Borrowed Time

*Artificial Organs and the
Politics of Extending Lives*

Health, Society, and Policy,
a series edited by Sheryl Ruzek and Irving Kenneth Zola

Borrowed Time

Artificial Organs and the Politics of Extending Lives

ALONZO L. PLOUGH

Temple University Press

PHILADELPHIA

To the memory of my father

Temple University Press, Philadelphia 19122
© 1986 by Temple University. All rights reserved
Published 1986
Printed in the United States of America

Library of Congress Cataloging-in-Publication Data

Plough, Alonzo L.
  Borrowed time.

  (Health, society, and policy)
  Includes index.
  1. Renal insufficiency—Treatment—Government policy—
United States.   2. Renal insufficiency—Treatment—Social
aspects—United States.   3. Technology assessment—
United States.   I. Title.   II. Series.   [DNLM: 1. Ethics,
Medical—United States.   2. Financing, Government—
economics—United States.   3. Health Policy—United
States.   4. Kidney Failure, Chronic—therapy.
WJ 342 P731b]
RA645.R35P55   1986   362.1'97461   85-26196
ISBN 0-87722-415-3

The paper used in this publication meets the minimum requirements of
American National Standard for Information Sciences—Permanence of Paper for Printed Library Materials, ANSI Z39.48-1984

Contents

Acknowledgments

I want to express a special thanks to my teachers at Cornell, where I was fortunate to pursue an unusual course of training for an anthropologist. Ken Kennedy's encouragement to stretch the application of medical anthropology was extremely important. Sandy Kelman's lessons on the political economy of health provided the practical focus for my developing interest in American medicine. Rose Goldsen inspired me to develop a critical view of the role of mass media as a force in public policy.

I am indebted to members of the Department of Epidemiology and Public Health of the Yale medical school, where I made the transition from a general interest in health to a professional focus on health policy. George Rosen, Arthur Viseltier, and especially Lowell Levin grounded my interests in the tradition of public health. A grant from the Center for Health Studies at Yale allowed me to conduct part of the research for this book. I owe a special thanks to Donald Riedell for this research support.

Most of the research on which this book is based was conducted at the University Health Policy consortium, a collaboration of Boston University, Brandeis University, and The Massachusetts Institute of Technology. While there I received grant support from the Health Care Financing Administration of the U.S. Department of Health and Human Services (18-p97038/1-05). I was fortunate to work with some special and talented people on these series of studies. Susanne Salem provided both insights and an attention to detail that resulted in work that exceeded our expectations. Michael Shwartz provided a rigorous structure for inquiry into the complex problems of medical technology. His probing analysis and intellectual energy greatly increased my understanding of the issues discussed in this work.

I am grateful for the collaborative efforts of the staff at the Michigan Kidney Registry that provided the data for the case-mix studies. Jack Weller provided important clinical insights from the perspective of a nephrologist, and Bill Ferguson assisted in data management.

Others who provided helpful comments during the course of this work include Harry Marks, Jonathan Brown, Susan Bell, Rosemary Taylor, Susan Reverby, Margert Gertise, Evan Stark, Ralph Berry, Jeff Prottas, Paul Eggers, Cathy Reissman, C. R. Blagg, Merry Minkler, Sandy Schwartz, and Allen Dyer.

I want to thank Ann Gerroir and Arville Grady, who survived multiple drafts and a new word processing program to provide a final manuscript, and Michael Arnott, who provided valuable research assistance during the final stage of manuscript preparation.

My greatest debt is to the patients, families, and staff of the renal unit where I learned first-hand the complexities, tragedies, and triumphs encountered in the treatment of end-stage renal disease. While I am sure that some of them will not agree entirely with my presentation and interpretation of their experiences, I hope that I have captured some of the important issues that confront the treatment of this catastrophic illness.

Finally, Jeanette Valentine has supported this project from the very first glimmer of ideas to the completion of the book. Throughout it all her insights, sage counsel, and clear logic have made this a better book. I thank her, and our son Louis, for what was, in many ways, our collective labor.

Parts of this book have been adapted from previously published articles of mine. The following materials have been reprinted by permission: Alonzo L. Plough, "Medical Technology and the Crisis of Experience: The Cost of Clinical Legitimation," *Social Science and Medicine* (Pergamon Press) 15F (1981): 89–101; Alonzo L. Plough and S. R. Salem, "Social and Contextual Factors in the Analysis of Mortality in End-Stage Renal Disease Patients," *American Journal of Public Health* 72 (1982): 1293–95; A. Plough, M. Shwartz, and S. Salem, "Greater Efficiency or Case-Mix Differences?: Fact vs. Fantasy in ESRD Reimbursement Policy," *Dialysis and Trans-*

plantation 13, no. 10 (Oct. 1984): 8–18; A. L. Plough, S. R. Salem, M. Shwartz et al., "Case-Mix in End-Stage Renal Disease: Differences between Patients in Hospital-Based and Free-Standing Treatment Facilities," *New England Journal of Medicine* 310 (1984): 1432–36; Alonzo Plough et al., "Severity Analysis in End-Stage Renal Disease: A Risk Group Approach," *ASAIO* (American Society for Artificial Internal Organs) *Journal* 8, no. 1 (Jan.–March 1985): 33–40.

Borrowed Time

*Artificial Organs and the
Politics of Extending Lives*

INTRODUCTION

The Social Context
of Medical Miracles

This book examines a dramatic medical technology, the treatment of kidney failure. "Those who would have died before now live" is the hallmark effect of a medical success, and the technologies that treat kidney failure are associated with such medical miracles. The case of kidney failure, called end-stage renal disease (ESRD) by clinical experts, has an important role in the development of federal policies toward life-extending technologies and the public perception of the technological fix in medicine. First of all, the technologies used to treat kidney failure (dialysis, called the "artificial kidney," and kidney transplantation) are the only extreme medical technologies that the government subsidizes as an entitlement for all those who require them to live. Second, the public as well as many medical practitioners no longer view kidney dialysis and transplantation as unusual or extreme procedures. *Newsweek*, in a December 1984 feature article on the artificial heart, called the use of the artificial kidney a "commonplace procedure" and noted that twenty years ago it was considered a highly emotional public issue, as the use of the artificial heart is now, but that today it is a routine practice. Is kidney failure a solved problem because over 70,000 persons receive federally subsidized treatment at a cost of nearly $2 billion a year? Or is the procedure routine because it has become more difficult to confront the many social and technological problems that remain under the surface of this designated medical miracle?

I chose to look at this particular example of a medical technology, the treatment of kidney failure, to make some general points about American medicine, the problem of chronic and catastrophic illness, and the cultural and political forces that have come to shape the current and future development of policies concerning new technologies. Why kidney failure? Is this not so focused and specialized a problem that it cannot be used as a general example of political and cultural issues in American medicine? These are fair questions. In this book I will analyze the way that the development of the artificial kidney and kidney transplantation set the stage for the development of a panoply of related technologies that are only now in the earliest stages of clinical application. In fact, the artificial kidney and the artificial heart were invented by the same biomedical researcher and represent a continuity of a clinical dream, the totally replaceable body. Artificial organs and organ transplantation are key symbols of American medicine's progress against death.

Recent transplantation activity in liver, heart, pancreas, lung, and other complex human organs and the development of artificial organs like the artificial heart together raise a number of important clinical, ethical, and political questions. These questions were raised initially in the early stages of kidney dialysis and transplantation. Examples include: Are these technologies experimental or tested therapies? Can society really afford to provide such miracles for all in need? Will there be widespread use of the technology if the government pays the bill? What are the issues concerning the quality of life for persons who must depend on these machines to survive? Will the profit-making firms take over? If so, with what effect on access, quality, and costs?

The treatment of kidney failure is often considered to be an example of the successful resolution of at least some of these vexing questions. Yet a close look at ESRD technologies in use and at the federal program that attempts to manage the costs and quality of these treatments suggests that most of these serious problems remain, although they are not dramatically publicized. Technical and ethical dilemmas have been transformed into a series of hidden problems; tragic choices continue to be made—not overtly, but through a system of silent triage. Policy makers never see treatment realities, only the promise of the medical miracle and, later, the price tag that is always higher than expected.

This book looks beneath the veneer of slightly tarnished success and demonstrates that the problem of kidney failure has been obscured rather than solved. Public subsidization of the clinical use of the technologies of dialysis and transplantation have instead created another set of problems, larger in scale and yet more difficult to see. The federal entitlements force the rationing of services in subtle but important ways. Survival and rehabilitation depend as much on the social class of the patient as on the miracle of the technology. The cure is not a cure but a prolongation of life, and the quality of those prolonged months or years ranges from pure agony to remarkable adjustment. The technical spectacle is given undue emphasis and comes to symbolize a clinical promise that is rarely fulfilled for patients or their care providers.

How do we differentiate between the miracle and the mirage in modern medicine? These are the hidden dimensions of a technical intervention that must be looked at closely. I will argue throughout this book that only through a comprehensive understanding can technologies like the artificial kidney or heart and the transplantation of livers, kidneys, or lungs be fairly assessed. The usual approach to technology assessment in medicine involves the quantitative analysis of technical data on survival, costs, and benefits of a particular technology. This research tradition has enshrined a form of "objective" study (exemplified by the randomized clinical trial) that is supposed to tell us which technologies are worth public investment. Then the economists overlay a cost-benefit analysis on the clinical assessment of the technology. As a result, we choose the variables that are easiest to measure (length of survival or cost of the procedure) and base most of our evaluation on these data. This form of technology assessment will, as a general rule, ignore the hidden dimensions of contradiction and conflict in the variety of experiences that people have with a medical technology.

In this book I present an alternative to the conventional way medical technology is evaluated. My approach is based on a set of analytic maxims that correct what I consider to be the myopia inherent in the more typical study of a medical technology. We must understand the actual experiences with these technologies in the lives of real patients. There are resounding success stories and chronicles of fates worse than death. We must question with heightened skepticism the received knowledge of clinical science and ask what are the social and ethical assumptions of the ideal of the totally replaceable body. Do we see a transplantation of health care priorities? We must try to understand the mixture of compassion and hubris that has come to typify high-technology medicine. We must comprehend the growing role of profit-making firms in high-technology medicine and push our analysis beyond simplistic notions of competition and efficiency. Finally, we are obligated to look beyond the "objective" domain of scientific analysis of outcomes that are relatively simple to measure. It is essential to understand the cultural context of our fear of death and our hopes for technological control over the uncertainties of living and dying.

I look within these dimensions of the experience and analysis of medical technology in the chapters that follow. I chose the case study of kidney failure to provide a focused and detailed description of the whole range of problems encountered in the use of extreme medical technologies like artificial organs and organ transplantation. Such a format allows me to juxtapose contrasting views, to expose contradictions, and, simply, to tell a story that highlights the varieties of experience with a particular disease. Through this approach we can begin to see the pattern that connects the seemingly unrelated domains of culture, technology, policy, and the experience of illness. I offer this as a framework through which we might come to better understand the technological imperative in medicine.

My frame of reference is similar to that of Richard Titmuss in his book *The Gift Relationship*. Titmuss used the example of public policies for the collection and distribution of human blood to address a larger social issue: the role of altruism versus the profit motive in the design of public policy. Through the detailed study of the case of blood policy, he spoke to broad and important issues of justice, ethics, and the orientating philosophy of the welfare state. What kind of society do we want and which principles best guide the vision of a just and equitable state? These are the questions that concerned him over ten years ago and that are even more critical today.

The book is divided into two parts. The four chapters of Part I describe how patients, families, and clinicians come to hold widely different and even contradictory definitions of the problems of kidney failure. Each group experiences this illness in a different way and, as a result, holds different expectations about the disease and the technologies used to treat it. There are, in fact, different relationships with the technology and conflicting notions of success and failure.

The introduction to Part I presents a theoretical background for the chapters that follow. My concern here is to present a framework that sees medicine as more than just a set of technologies to combat death and disability. It is also a way of thinking about life and death. This way of thinking has a history, incorporates ritual, cherishes certain beliefs, develops elaborate rites of passage, and defines other competing frameworks as taboo. In short, medicine can be viewed as a *culture* where life-extending technologies like organ transplantation play a key symbolic role. Even more importantly, medicine is also a part of a broader culture, a collective Western consciousness, where the notion of progress through the technological control of nature is a bedrock belief. The cultural authority of medicine derives from its ability to tap into this bedrock of hope in technological mastery. Dramatic life-extending technologies like kidney dialysis seem to legitimate the profession's claim to be a repository of hope against the uncertainties of life and death.

The reader who is less interested in theory or prefers to examine the data first would be advised to begin with Chapter 1, where the analysis of the case of kidney failure starts. Chapter 1 begins with a brief history of the development of nephrology (the study of the kidney) and the technologies used to treat kidney failure; it continues with a presentation and interpretation of basic data on treatment outcomes and the clinical controversies in nephrology. The focus in this chapter is on the ways doctors construct a framework through which they define success and failure in clinical terms. It is a study of the ideas that shape the context of ESRD treatment. I raise two questions central to the analysis of the problem of kidney failure and the broader implications of this study: Is there a characteristic logic to the practice of medicine that oversimplifies human-scale crisis? Does this oversimplification contribute to the dilemmas of federal policy toward medical technology and to the increase in private market involvement in high-technology medicine?

Chapter 2 focuses on the social dynamics of problem solving in ESRD treatment, the effect the clinical way of knowing has on the illness experience. The clinical framework of nephrologists narrows the wide-ranging complexity of kidney failure to create a more manageable construction of the disease. The data drawn from nearly two years of participant-observation research in an ESRD treatment program includes interviews with patients and their families, doctors, nurses, and others who provide care for them. It also includes excerpts from staff meetings where patients were discussed, problems raised, and tensions aired. The chapter provides a revealing look at the experience of medical uncertainty and suggests that clinical theory provides an inadequate problem-solving context in ESRD treatment for both practitioners and patients.

In Chapter 3 I examine how health care professionals can, simultaneously, recognize the limitations of their clinical frameworks and exacerbate those conflicts in the pursuit of what they would call psychosocial remedies. Psychologists, social workers, and other professionals would describe themselves as providing a framework for the problems of kidney failure that differs from, and corrects for, the clinical perspective of nephrologists. I argue here that they are doctors in spite of themselves and label the patient's experience rather than provide an understanding of it.

Chapter 4 turns to a detailed look at the illness experience of two patients as expressed in their own terms. This is a movement away from the technological definition of illness in clinical terms and toward an understanding of the hopes, fears, aspirations, and concerns of people living with a more acute awareness of mortality than do the rest of us. The central concern of this chapter is to understand how patients struggle against the labels and frameworks for the experience that is thrust on them by the clinicians. They develop their own assessment of the technologies that extend their lives. We would make much more informed decisions about the use of extreme medical technologies if these voices could be heard.

Part II of the book returns to the larger social issues of medical technology in the American cultural context. The focus of the last three chapters is on the issues of economic costs, federal policies, and corporate involvement, the rhetoric of market efficiency and technical fixes that have come to dominate health policy in general and ESRD policy in particular.

The introduction to Part II describes the great conceptual and experiential gulf that separates living and dying with kidney failure and federal policies developed to manage the use of dialysis and transplantation. The nuances of patients' experiences with medical technology get lost in the policy makers' desire to control costs. Data are collected to monitor program outcomes in ESRD treatment, but even the most apparently simple measures, like mortality rates, mask a set of complex social problems.

Chapter 5 discusses the development of federal policy for ESRD and its impact on the organization of clinical treatment for kidney failure. How does the government regulate medical uncertainty? I look at the history of the ESRD reimbursement program with a particular focus on the assumptions behind a federal policy that provided an opportunity for the growth of profit-making dialysis clinics.

Chapter 6 moves to another powerful framework through which kidney failure is viewed: the market construction of disease. I will examine the development of the kidney business and the ways firms carve out lucrative opportunities from their experiences with medical technology. The firms that manufacture dialysis equipment and the firms that provide for-profit dialysis cherish the symbol of efficiency. Yet their business practices tend to increase the cost of ESRD treatment. This chapter is an extensive analysis of a series of problems suggested in the last chapter of Paul Starr's recent book, *The Social Transformation of American Medicine*: How do corporations shape the definition of health policy problems and, therefore, influence how the government funds programs to respond to these problems?

Chapter 7 considers the political economy of health services research in ESRD treatment. Research findings can influence a corporation's bottom line in the medical technology area. In fact, studies that evaluate the costs of a technology have both empirical and ideological dimensions; the assumptions about costs and efficiency condition the design and interpretation of the research. I look at the cost debate in ESRD and present an example of a particular corporation's attempt to prevent the publication of research findings that challenged the myth of market efficiency.

The Epilogue brings together all of the chapters, emphasizing their common themes: the varieties of hope invested in new machines (medical technologies), the nature of medical rhetoric, the power of medical mythology, and the effects of these forces on our experience of health and illness.

The book is unusual in its approach and develops a framework that some readers will not expect. In fact, many of the traditional paradigms for the analysis of medicine and technology are criticized. The "bottom line" of my analysis does not offer nostrums of conventional policy analysis, although there are clearly programmatic implications from this analysis. It is, primarily, an ethnographic study that uses a variety of methods to elucidate the culture of medical technology. The study does not design a way out of the dilemmas I describe. It is what Clifford Geertz calls "thick description"—a highly detailed description of our own conflicting experiences with extreme medical technology. The case study of kidney failure is diverse enough to support the range of questions necessary to explore the hidden problems of the technical fix in medicine.

PART I

On the Culture of Medicine and the Experience of Technology

How do we experience medical technology? What do these elaborate symbols of medical knowledge mean, and how do they shape our expectations of life and death? Obviously there are multiple forms of this experience and a diverse set of public expectations.[1] It might seem odd to think about medical technology as experience or as influenced by the meanings attached to it. Technology is closely related to another powerful frame of human experience and meaning: science. As such, we often think of technologies as representations or symbols of the rational force of science.[2] Public perceptions of medical technology are of highly complex machines or procedures that apply the power of science in our lives. Technologies are in the realm of "hard" approaches to human problems that appear somewhat separate from the more fragile uncertainties of everyday life. In illness, we often look to medical technologies to restore a lost sense of order, both biological and social, to our lives.

Our experience of medical technology is a personal knowledge derived from either participation or observation. The meaning of medical technology is derived from that which is signified or conveyed by such experiences. In American medicine the effectiveness of doctors' technological tool kit helps to establish the power of the profession as a whole. The technologies largely determine the profession's authority, the public's acceptance of medicine's scientific legitimacy.[3] As a result, the complex web of diverse experiences and different meanings attached to this powerful component of modern medical practice offers a view into the cultural dynamics of medicine.

I develop a framework for understanding the cultural dynamics of medicine by looking through the window of the experience of medical technology. Like all cultural institutions, medicine consists of ritual activities (practice) and rhetoric (persuasive accounts of those activities). I will focus on the many layers of symbols through which the cultural components of medicine are expressed and, in particular, on the persuasive accounts of medical ritual. How the ambiguous or uncertain medical technologies are presented (accounted for) in mass culture, and the social and political implications of the scientific rhetoric surrounding these technologies, are the central concerns of this book.

One way to narrow the range of this problem is to focus on one example of an uncertain and ambiguous medical technology: the treatment of kidney failure, most often referred to as "end-stage renal disease" (ESRD). The treatment of ESRD involves a very elaborate medical ritual that generates multiple levels of meaning through a variety of public and private experiences with the technologies of dialysis and transplantation. These levels of experience include the person with kidney failure, the family and social network around that person, the medical care providers who treat the patient's disease, the clinical researchers who develop a scientific framework for the disease process, the federal bureaucrats who regulate payment for ESRD treatment, the private firms that make up the ESRD business, and, finally, the public understanding derived from observation and primarily through the media. To begin, I will sketch here the general problem medicine poses for cultural understanding of technology and health.

What Are the Cultural Dynamics of Medicine?

The critical study of medicine as a social institution has generated almost two decades of intense analysis, ranging from the descriptive reports of the "American Health Empire" to more detailed political theories of the power of medicine under capitalism.[4] Throughout these diverse critiques, there is one repeated point: medicine is a scientifically based technique that has gone astray. For example, one of the primary critical assessments of medicine sees it as socially unresponsive, captured by the political and economic forces of capitalism.[5] Other social critiques damn medicine for not being effective, and a flurry of writings across the political spectrum demand demonstrations—through statistics and clinical trials—that medicine be proven effective, that there be more truth in the social packaging of its products.[6] Insurance companies encourage second opinions of diagnoses, and practitioners push forward "improved" alternatives for treating various maladies. There is an ironic sense of disappointment about medicine's failure to deliver the goods, even in the most extreme charges by critics. Sociologists and others have raised another set of problems about medicine. They have argued that there has been an expansion of the illness category beyond the demonstrable organic pathology of the body. Thus, the label of illness becomes a strategy of social control with moral and punitive connotations.[7] Bluntly put, the social problem is one of monitoring this encroachment into the labeling of normative social activity.

And so it goes. Numerous studies conclude that medicine ignores social contexts, is not rationally organized, is sexist, racist, and elitist.[8] We also have discovered that certain medical technologies are, indeed, effective, although understanding the social context of a medical success is far from straightforward.

Most of the prevailing critiques of medicine embrace a central strategy whose goal is to revise and capture, for useful social purposes, the control of medical care and its technology. While this is politically important in the short run and provides a focus for an activist strategy, it does not clearly address the cultural problems of medicine.

In order to develop a cultural critique, we need to go beyond medicine's role *in* our culture to an understanding of medicine *as* a culture. We need to understand the nuances, orientations, standards for knowledge, what concepts are held to be negotiable, and which are considered inviolable, as well as medicine's framework for self-justification.

In short, an examination of the cultural dynamics of medicine is an interpretative study in search of what the anthropologist Clifford Geertz has called "webs of significance."[9] The task is to understand how medicine provides a context in which public consciousness about health and illness is generated. As the French social historian Michel Foucault shows in *The Birth of the Clinic*, medicine has developed a perspective in which certain events and not others become certifiable problems. The concept of the clinical gaze (how medicine looks at problems) is discussed by Foucault. His analysis attempts to discover the conditions through which particular illness experiences are structured into a way of viewing that maintains itself through the generalized form we could call a clinical paradigm. The gaze ostensibly selects truth, but it in fact creates its own version of experience and formally organizes a language around it. It is a "truth that they owe not to light, but to the slowness of the gaze that passes over them, around them, and into them, bringing them nothing more than its own light."[10] This is not a gaze that reduces, it is one that establishes, defines, and structures, in this case, the domain of medical culture.

Rituals and Rhetoric

In the ritual (practice) of medicine the overwhelming emphasis on technology has created many problems, ranging from questions of ethics to issues of cost control. Much of the conventional analysis of these concerns focuses exclusively on the ritual and ceremonial order of medicine, examining such topics as doctor-patient relationships and conflicts, ineffective or harmful medical procedures, and the emphasis of treatment over prevention. Although these concerns are extremely important outcomes of the culture of medicine, the narrowness of this practice-oriented inquiry largely limits critiques to analyses of what medical professionals do or do not do within clinical contexts or in direct extensions of those contexts. And frameworks that see medicine only as a "wayward science" or simply "unresponsive technology" are derived from this ritual-centered focus. Some critics would go so far as to say that medicine is not sufficiently scientific (objective) and that this is the cause of these problems.[11] Uncritical assumptions about the scientific principles underlying medical practice are dormant within this perspective.

The scientific ideal in the practice of medicine is in itself a major issue for analysis. The problem of the quest for scientific ideals in medicine forms a conceptual bridge that connects the ritual of medicine to an understanding of the rhetoric (persuasive accounts) of medicine. The problem is the tension between medicine's role as a science that discovers a predictive set of laws about the nature and treatment of disease and medicine's role in the clinical application of scientific knowledge, where social, political, and personal experience confound the predictive regularity of medical events.

The rhetoric of medicine involves the use of scientifically pre-sented "facts" to provide a compelling argument for the ritual of medicine. It is perhaps more a part of the framework for the justifica-tion of rituals than a guide for medical practice. The scientific accounts found within medical rhetoric present the framework for what can be "said" and categories through which legitimate versions of the medical story can be told. For example, viral or genetic causes for cancer form a more acceptable accounting for the etiology of this disease in medical culture than factors such as work or stress. Specific clinical defects are more "logical" than social or cultural determinants of illness. Such accounts form an important part of the expressive culture of medicine and provide the basis of a system for claiming authority and justifying its power. Persuasive accounts present an apparently ordered world of medical facts and health problems in a way that is calculated to induce the lay public to believe in medicine's technical prowess. An important characteristic of medical rhetoric is the way that these accounts provide a framework that appears to be internally valid and unambiguous and, hence, has no need for exter-nal (public) justification. Thus, the rhetorical framework of medicine establishes both a public meaning about the role of medicine in society *and* a reference through which we filter personal and social experiences of health and illness. Joseph Gusfield, in his book *The Culture of Public Problems*, recognized the hidden power that such accounts carry:

> The most subtle forms of social control are those we least recognize as such. Precisely because the categories of understanding and meaning provide so powerful a constraint to what we experience and how we think about that experience, they prevent awareness of alternative ways of conceiving events and processes. Because they lead us to "see" the accustomed forms as the only reality they minimize and obscure the possible conflicts and the voluntary decisions that have helped construct that "reality."[12]

The cultural dynamics of medicine shape our perception of health or illness through both ritual and rhetoric. A form of knowledge is advanced, and a manner of expressing that knowledge, which has the potential to be separate from, and often counter to, social or personal understandings of illness and health. By selectively recognizing tech-nical problems that are oriented toward technical solutions, we dis-miss alternative ways of framing health and illness (socially, politically, or through personal experience) as marginal or less significant concerns. Nonetheless, these alternative paradigms for health and illness have a potential force to create dissonance within the core tenets of medical culture. Voices from these alternative frameworks struggle to overcome both the explicit constraints of ritual (doctor-patient interactions) and the more subtle barriers of rhetoric (public notions of the success of technical medicine) in order to express a different context in which the meaning of health and illness can be examined in our own lives. Many voices are unsuccessful. Most of us accept the definitions of health found in the orthodox medical rhetoric because it seems to reflect a formidable and seemingly impenetrable self-justifying system. This is especially so because most of us usually are ill, and hence in a vulnerable position, when we think about medicine—a situation in which giving in often seems to be prudent.

Media Accounts—Reporting the Culture of Medicine on Its Own Terms

Persuasive rhetorical accounts do not just happen; they must be continuously updated, embellished, and maintained. To have apparent validity, such accounts must also respond to political and economic conditions and, to some extent, public sentiment. The expressive component of the culture of medicine articulates these changing accounts—not always, however, within those settings and activities we would call clinical.

The representation of medicine and health in the public media (newspapers, TV, movies) is an important component of social life that influences our understanding and experience of illness. The media expand and dramatize medical problems and contribute to the social process of how isolated "facts" emerge later as a "public" problem. This occurs in many forms and in complex, even contradictory ways. The issue of medicine and the media goes far beyond the problem of imprecise, or even misleading, reporting. While sensationalism and the reduction of complex issues to "lifestyle" stories characterize much of medical reporting, the culture of medicine also supports this tendency. The simple technical fix of developing more scientifically trained medical writers would have limited influence on the representational problems of medicine and the public media.

Journalistic accounts of the culture of medicine induce beliefs about events or problems that we may not experience personally but that we share publicly as an aggregate form of "knowing." They present images of medical problems that are "fatal" or "tragic," "serious" or "not serious," and "known" or "speculative." This is an important part of the cultural organization of medicine and the constitution of the meanings of health and illness in everyday life. An important issue here is how these journalistic accounts present areas of uncertainty within medicine such as new medical technologies.

There are, of course, a number of explicitly ambiguous and uncertain areas of medical culture. These are categories or problems that are difficult to manage with the usual rituals and rhetoric. One of the most dramatic of these is chronic illness, which poses a set of conditions that typify the tensions and stresses within the culture of medicine. The treatment of chronic illness (cancer, heart disease, diabetes, etc.) is the source of many of medicine's public problems. Cost control, the appropriateness of certain technologies, and ethical dilemmas all play a large part in the story of chronic illness.

Clinical approaches to chronic illness characteristically apply medical technologies to highly uncertain diseases. And many social problems that can result from this technologically dominated approach are evident most clearly in the dynamics of the experience of illness itself. Therapeutic solutions, however, attempt to define health problems by setting technical boundaries and through this largely redefine the social components of the medical problem. The ritual of medicine is presented as being responsible for success, which, in turn, is defined as the technical effectiveness of treatment; failure, where it occurs, is largely attributed to the individual deficiencies of "unsuccessful" patients. Ambiguity, of course, is downplayed. And this is echoed in the press.

For example, let us return to one chronic illness, kidney failure (ESRD), about which reports in the media present a reality that is at best partial and at worst misleading. ESRD is clinically defined as a biological situation where the kidneys do not function and where this condition is irreversible and permanent. This is a chronic disease that requires treatment by dialysis (three times a week, six hours a treatment) or kidney transplantation. In the United States this is the only chronic illness for which a federal program (since 1972) pays virtually all treatment costs. Almost $2 billion (1985) is expended on medical technologies for ESRD. The technical approach dominates the care of this chronic illness, providing a clear example of the "technical fix." The technology maintains the patient in the disease. It prevents immediate death at the same time that it provides a highly variable and sometimes problematic quality of life.

When the government began payment for this condition, nephrology "came of age," said the prestigious *New England Journal of Medicine* in a presentation of the internal rhetoric of the culture of medicine.[13] How was this successful coming of age (rite of passage) accounted for to the public?

As early as 1962 *Life* magazine focused national attention on the the moral frame of dialysis. Shana Alexander's article "They Decide Who Lives and Who Dies: Medical Miracle Puts Moral Burden on Small Committee" is characteristic of the way the press examines new medical technology by combining "gee-whiz" reporting with a sketch of the obvious ethical question of a technological "choice" for life and death.[14] The story is of tragic choices and powerful technologies that give life if a patient is fortunate enough to be selected. The message is that frail human selection committees have to say no because resources are scarce and all in need cannot receive this gift of life. The meta-message is that technologies give life, that any clinically defined judgment of meaningful extension of life is a social good, and that there should be broader access to medical miracles. Thus a public problem emerges from accounts like this of the new technology: ought not the government pay for this gift of life for all in need?

A powerful image of medical technology is represented through such reporting frames. The machine becomes a symbol of life against death, and the technology, therefore, offers deliverance. A peculiar notion of equity is introduced that considers equal access to medical miracles a moral imperative. At the same time, any larger issues of social justice are not part of this imperative; there is a narrow right to technologically mediated life. Inequality becomes an issue of public morality only at the precipice of death.

The journalistic frame of the "medical miracle" dominated the early reporting of ESRD during the 1960s and early 1970s. Many articles in the mass media described the "tragic choices" made by selection committees and the need for public funds to assist in the ethical allocation of medical technologies.[15] This early period represents a critical historical moment when the newly emerged technology of dialysis began to take on a powerful symbolic role in the rhetoric of medical culture. This was the first artificial organ that could be represented as a success. The totally implantable artificial heart had developed a public track record as a failure in the early 1970s. In fact, the obviously experimental nature of the artificial heart proved to be an embarrassment to surgeons, like Denton Cooley, who in 1973 attempted premature therapeutic applications.[16]

As in the case of the space program, the miracle technologies of medicine represented a symbol of progress into a new frontier. Such Promethean examples of human mastery over the unknown and feared domains of inner and outer space are culturally quite powerful. The images and stories presented in the media tap into the core metaphors through which we give meaning to life and attempt to deny the certainty of death. Hence, the power of the technology is borrowed, at least in part, from deeply rooted cultural symbols of hope and deliverance, literally for a *deus ex machina*.

"Dialysis or Death" began a 1974 *New York Times Magazine* article.[17] It reported that "some 16,000 kidney failure victims are alive because of one of the most successful medical experiments ever."[18] Ten years after the first public representation of ESRD, the images of deliverance are still being reinforced. Profiled in this article is "an attractive young woman in her middle 20's who watches TV, eats a meal she had prepared, and does dialysis at home. Without the regular assistance of this machine [she] would, in a matter of weeks, die."[19] Although this journalistic account recognizes that not all dialysis patients are "bouncing with energy," the successful patient is emphasized (given voice).[20] The image of mastery over death is prominent, and any problems with this technologically mediated life are only marginal concerns.

When the problems of medical technologies are discussed in the press, they are presented in a narrow and fragmented manner. The impression is that there is no generic problem with the medical technology, simply a set of partial problems. In the case of ESRD these problem fragments include such things as the cost of the technology or issues in the availability of alternatives to dialysis—all, matters of increasing efficiency. Cost issues are represented in the press by such titles as "Kidney Care Plan's Cost Soars" or "Concern Rising Over Costs of Kidney Dialysis Program."[21] In one form or another, these articles state that we spend billions of public dollars for this condition and ask, are there more rational approaches to regulation?

"Transplants Shortage of Donors Still Acute" and the three-part series "Alternatives to Kidney Dialysis" discuss the possibilities of the more "effective" technology of transplantation.[22] Here the problem is simply defined as a lack of enough kidneys to transplant. Effectiveness is defined as a lower initial cost for transplantation compared with dialysis. The shift in the orienting frame of these stories reflects a concern with "market ethics"—the moral imperative of cost control. This represents a later stage in the public story of ESRD, when the metaphors begin to become mixed.

An example of this shift in the orientation of media accounts of this disease is an article entitled "Economics of Life and Death Arises in Debate Over Rising Kidney Therapy."[23] Here another successful patient is profiled:

At 5:30, he put down his papers at the Justice Department, where he works as a lawyer, and hopped into his new rust-colored Toyota Supra.

Without delay, the 35-year-old Mr. Schoen headed for Holy Cross Hospital in suburban Silver Spring, MD. He parked, walked purposefully into a basement room, sat down in a big blue armchair, and held his left arm out on a pillow. A therapist plunged two huge 16 gauge needles into his arm, one into an artery and the other into a vein. Moments later, his wine-red blood was filtering through a dialyzer that does the cleansing job that his kidneys had quit doing for him nearly 10 years ago.

Soon the Bronx-born lawyer was leaning back, munching on Dorito chips and leafing through the newspaper. Three and one-quarter hours later, he was unhooked and headed home, feeling better. It is a routine he goes through every Monday, Wednesday, and Friday evening.[24]

The writer profiled an employed professional man who is supposed to represent an average patient on dialysis. His illness is presented as a relatively minor annoyance to his active work life. But this does not represent the experience of the majority of patients who have kidney failure. A less public study published in the *New England Journal of Medicine* demonstrated that only 25 percent of ESRD patients are able to hold a job outside their home because of their illness.[25]

The following chapters will suggest that the experience of kidney failure for most patients is far from the routine presented in most "human interest"-oriented media accounts. Rather, it involves establishing a tentative equilibrium between the physical, psychological, and social problems accompanying a debilitating chronic illness and the attempt to hold onto an integrated life outside of treatment. Patients are not kept alive indefinitely. (Only 30 percent of ESRD patients nationally survive longer than five years.[26]) Further, the relative effectiveness of different treatment modalities has not been demonstrated in an adequate study. With few exceptions, the reasons for long- or short-term survival by patients is poorly understood—reasons that involve social and economic as well as clinical factors.

The inappropriate assumptions in the media about the realities of treatment for ESRD obscure ethical issues and discount the experience of many patients who have suffered kidney failure. Hopeful accounts of successful middle-class professionals make good copy. The problem is that they also tend to present an impression to the public that most ESRD patients are healthy and active and employed. This sort of presentation—based on medical rhetoric rather than experience—is detrimental to the many ESRD patients who do have substantial problems. These patients, who do have to cope with complications and uncertainty, come to be viewed as examples of personal failure rather than as examples of the struggle against the generic limitations of the technological imperative in medicine.

Although there may be allusions to the complex dynamics of ESRD treatment and a recognition that some patients do not fare so well, the emphasis is always to return to the "success" stories, that is, to patients whose experience is consistent with medical rhetoric. Occasionally there is an anecdotal story of an obvious ethical problem, such as the proposed plan by a U.S. physician to purchase kidneys from living, indigent donors for sale to persons needing transplants. But this problem, as well as the continual concern with explicit rationing of resources for ESRD, only hints at the broader social and cultural dilemmas I will describe. What, then, are the problems in the shadows of the media frame that could inform our public understanding of the experience of medical technology? Part I of this book will present some of the political, social, and cultural problems that have been given little attention in media accounts.

What is the image and what is the reality in the culture of medicine? Clinical rhetoric in both media and internal professional accounts presents a highly selective vision of medical practice. Most new technologies are reported as "promising." Where uncertainty is noted, the successes are emphasized and the ambiguity of medical practices is moved to the background. Obvious ethical dilemmas are seen as bizarre and unconnected to inherent problems of the technical fix in medicine. The rhetoric is not completely false, but it is seriously unbalanced.

We have a problem here because our collective experience of medical technology is shaped, in large part, by media and other public accounts. Expectations concerning the experience of illness, the threat of death, and the role of medicine merge and become a public way of knowing—our common sense. Yet, when illness occurs as a personal event, when a medical technology is depended on for life, not just read about, a dissonance between private meaning and public accounts may arise. Even while one may be labeled a "successful" patient, there can be potential problems. When the label becomes more negative (chronic, terminal, difficult, etc.), it represents a manifest crisis—a battle over the meaning of illness in the course of one's life. As the following chapters will detail, this can become part of an uphill struggle waged in a context ordered by two of the dominant cultural metaphors of our time, the "logic" of science and the "efficiency" of the market. The culture of medicine, with its elaborate ritual and its powerful rhetoric, also struggles with these same metaphors.

CHAPTER ONE

Clinical Theory
The Conceptual Context of a Medical Practice

Many social problems result from a technology-dominated approach to the uncertainties of chronic illness and are clearly evident in the dynamics of the illness experience. The attempt to set technical boundaries for the definition of health problems largely defines away the social components of the illness. As a result, success is usually attributed to the effectiveness of treatment. Failure is often viewed as resulting from the individual deficiencies of unsuccessful patients. Both portrayals attempt to establish the effectiveness of a medical technology.

The central concern that this and the following two chapters address is the relationship among *medical uncertainty, the illness experience*, and the *characteristics of "objective" professional discourse*.

Clinical outcomes in ESRD demonstrate the problems of medical uncertainty. ESRD patients are very likely to have other diseases such as diabetes or hypertension, making treatment a highly complicated undertaking. The clinical account of the problem of ESRD can be described generally as an attempt to define *effectiveness* in a way that could set boundaries to these far-ranging problems. Effectiveness of treatment is therefore defined in dichotomous terms such as life versus death or renal function versus no renal function. Through this narrow definition of effectiveness, the limitations of current technologies in controlling the mortality and morbidity associated with ESRD are deemphasized. I will first present a very brief historical sketch of the development of the artificial kidney and kidney transplantation within nephrology. Then I will examine in some detail the clinical account of ESRD that emerges from the interaction of half-way technologies and ambiguous disease.

The Clinical Construction of ESRD

A brief review of the history of renal dialysis and transplantation indicates that the renal physician, or nephrologist, had a considerable professional stake in obtaining federal funding for ESRD treatment.[1] In interviews I conducted with federal officials involved with the ESRD program in the early years and with other physicians, the term *nephrology community* often came up. During the early 1960s when dialysis and transplantation remained explicitly experimental treatment modalities, those physicians involved with ESRD were viewed as somewhat marginal to the traditional medical community. As one federal official commented:

> Dialysis in the late 60's was a back-room enterprise. It was usually done off in an isolated corner in some dark part of the hospital. This caused the practicing nephrologists to become quite cliqueish as a group, and as a result, they established the coordination that allowed them to successfully lobby for research and treatment funds.[2]

The advent of federal funding for dialysis and transplantation represented a victory for those physicians who considered costs to be the major barrier to clinical breakthroughs in the treatment of chronic renal failure. A presumably neutral federal agency would allocate resources for treatment, making the problems of access to therapy and the painful decisions regarding who receives treatment appear to have been solved. Given this perspective, the only remaining problem for nephrologists was to devise a set of uniform criteria for the delivery of patient care services; a federally funded ESRD program would ensure that these services would be dispensed to all recipients in some standard and, ideally, cost-effective way.[3] The nephrology community interpreted the idea of equitable treatment under the law as a challenge to establish the *optimal* treatment modality among the clinical procedures available (transplantation, hemodialysis or peritoneal dialysis, and home versus in-center location of treatment). Thus, early on in the history of federally funded

ESRD care, the equity of access issue that was so vexing an ethical problem became a relative nonissue. The focus for the new governmentally supported physicians was to determine the best clinical approach to treatment.

The determination of the best or optimal mode of treatment proved not to be a simple or entirely objective process. Physicians differed widely in their choice of treatment for ESRD. The major difference was and continues to be between transplant surgeons and nephrologists; each group believes that its particular specialty provides a superior solution.[4]

Transplant surgeons generally consider dialysis as an interim measure that allows patients to survive until a suitable kidney is found for transplantation. The usefulness of dialysis is thus related only to the shortage of kidney donors. The early advocates of transplantation cited estimates that 15,000, or one-third of the 40,000 patients in this country receiving chronic kidney dialysis therapy in 1975, were on waiting lists for a kidney. The solution to the treatment problem, from this perspective, was to recruit more kidney donors from the general population.[5]

Treatment facilities tended to emphasize one approach to treatment over another. For example, at Boston's Brigham and Women's Hospital, where the first kidney transplant was conducted in 1954, more patients have received renal transplants than at any other facility in the world. The hospital proudly noted that a high percentage of its transplant patients return to productive work. The only exceptions are "those individuals exhibiting inadequate or dependent personalities. A few individuals even hold down several jobs!" This definition of a success linked transplantation with economically productive patient outcomes and failure with a psychological deficiency in the patient. I will examine the issue of the rehabilitation potential of ESRD patients later, but it is important to recognize that transplantation is viewed by its advocates as a cure, both clinically and socially.[6]

Advocates of dialysis countered this position by emphasizing the comparatively poor survival of cadaver transplants and the multiple complications that can follow immunosuppression therapy. This position was best represented by W. J. Kolff and Belding Scribner, both of whom were major figures in the original network of nephrologists who developed dialysis during the 1960s. For them, the optimal treatment of ESRD is dialysis (the artificial organ), and they predicted that in the future dialysis technology would eventually develop implantable artificial or bionic kidneys.[7]

This dispute between subspecialties (not an uncommon phenomenon in medicine) constitutes a special problem for the dynamics of ESRD treatment. A physician who was also a patient with ESRD commented on the effect of subspecialty tensions on patient care:

> The problem developed into the simple fact that the nephrologist and the transplant surgeon, within two different disciplines and ideologies, do not speak freely with one another to find "the true answer" for any individual patient. These specialists . . . work at odds, to the detriment of all their patients. And neither specialist informs or consults fully with the patient and his family about their needs and desires. The doctor is thus at a disadvantage of his own making—the terrible disadvantage of having knowledge of his patients' feelings about illness and treatment concealed from him.[8]

Although he recognized that there is an iatrogenic (physician-caused illness) outcome related to the emphasis of medical specialty interests over patient interests, he did not see this as an inherent problem of overspecialization and reification of the illness per se. Rather he, as many others, viewed the issue as a problem to be worked out within the medical model, and not as a problem that results from this model.

Prevention—The Unexamined Issue in the Clinical Model

Research into the etiology of the disease was seldom advanced during the development of ESRD theory in the early 1970s. Few studies to date have attempted to link etiological data into a representative model of the disease process.[9] (The complications related to ESRD treatment are quite extensive; pathological involvement of other organ systems is the rule rather than the exception.) When ESRD is considered within a broad social and biological framework, it becomes clear that current technologies provide relatively limited therapy. The focus on pathological renal tissue as the primary concern is quite consistent with the general orientation of the biomedical world. Progress and effectiveness become synonymous with better end-stage renal procedures that are evaluated on the basis of the simple dichotomies—renal function versus no renal function, life versus death. (Quality of life and an integrative social assessment of therapeutic interventions are not prominent considerations in the ideological premises of the technical fix.) Prevention is too hazy an issue for a profession that must rapidly contest for scientific legitimacy in the modern medical arena. Although some physicians find this trend lamentable, they are subjected to overwhelming pressure to refine the standard curative approaches rather than examine seriously approaches to prevention. Since they are continually faced with the identified, dying patient, such a response is understandable.

Clinical Studies—Patterns of the ESRD Problem

It would be an impossible task to review, even in summary, all of the relevant clinical literature in ESRD. This would also not serve well the purposes of this chapter. Instead, I want to describe (and try to make understandable to the general reader) the major technical and conceptual issues that emerge in the various reports, conferences, and journal articles by (mostly) physician investigators. This review is, therefore, somewhat selective, although it was based on a comprehensive computer-assisted search of the MEDLINE and MEDLARS data bases on ESRD from 1968 to 1985 encompassing over 500 separate entries.

There are other comprehensive assessments of the early history of renal technology. The various studies of Rettig and others provide a fascinating and detailed account of the development of dialysis by William Kolff during World War II and of the development in 1960 of the Quinton-Scribner shunt, which made maintenance dialysis possible.[10] I am less concerned here with the many factors influencing the actual decision by the federal government to fund the program. This will be considered in Part II of the book. The focus here is on the most visible documents of clinical problem definition and refinement since the passage of the federal funding program under Medicare in 1972. How have physicians shaped the contours of the ESRD problem? What are the central concerns? Who are the interest groups? What are the major contested dilemmas and nagging uncertainties of clinical theory in ESRD? In short, concern is with the organization of knowledge within the ESRD-oriented nephrology community; how do the people in this community choose to "own" this problem and, just as importantly, what do they choose to "disown"?

The locus of clinical concerns began to form recognizable and relatively stable categories during the mid-1970s. With the watershed of federal funding behind them and buoyed by the public understanding that dialysis and transplantation were no longer experiments but full-fledged therapies (although this distinction remains quite problematic on a conceptual level), those nephrologists constructing the clinical theory of ESRD faced a new set of problems. Perhaps the problems were not so new, as they were actually old problems in a changed social and political environment. Federal funding brought with it heightened public (or at least bureaucratic) scrutiny.

What was this program on which millions and soon billions of public dollars were being spent? The making of clinical theory in ESRD, then, was a multifold enterprise for nephrologists. In fact, and I will discuss this extensively in Part II, nephrology has increasingly had to share the forum of clinical problem definition with economists, ethicists, congressional committees, and others with health policy concerns. The boundaries of clinical theory were proving to be at least as permeable as the cellophane membranes of the artificial kidney; there were significant and not always controlled flows back and forth between the domains of clinical science and bureaucratic imperatives.

Certainly it would be an overstatement to define the period between 1973 and 1978 as a "state of siege" for nephrologists, but there was consistent pressure to produce and refine clinical knowledge in such a way that identifiable public concerns might be addressed. Conversely, the growing number of public forums (the media, Congress, agencies making health policy) thrust the relatively newly emerged ESRD clinicians into a more visible role than might be expected from a group of clinical scientists.

As late as 1977, we find in the *New England Journal of Medicine* a summing up of this clinical rite of passage in an editorial entitled "Nephrology Comes of Age." Written as a review of and reflection on the first seventeen years of the specialty of nephrology, it neatly chronicles the confident and optimistic self-perception of nephrologists during this time. Even as the political and economic environment around the new renal technologies was shifting, the clinical voice of authority presented a rather removed assessment of past accomplishment and future aspirations:

There was, in fact, little about nephrology in 1960 that would have defined it as a major clinical specialty and even less that would have predicted its astonishing subsequent growth. Nineteen sixty was the year in which the Quinton-Scribner shunt was described, but the efficacy of chronic hemodialysis in the management of end-stage renal disease had not yet been demonstrated. Renal transplantation was still in its infancy. Except for isografts between identical twins, the operation could then only be described as experimental—too hazardous for routine clinical application. Nephrology was therefore mainly the province of anatomists, physiologists and (especially after the advent of renal biopsy) pathologists, who were interested primarily in the structure and function of the kidney in health and disease.[11]

By the time of the third triennial meeting of the International Society of Nephrology, held in 1966, the situation had changed. Transplantation and hemodialysis were burgeoning and were beginning to transform the practice of renal medicine. Nephrology was changing from a gloomy clinical sideline for a few internists or pediatricians, on the one hand, or the arcane province of some clinical physiologist, on the other, to *"the self-proliferating giant it has now become."*[12] In discussing a meeting of American nephrologists in 1977 and prospects for the future, the writer notes:

Once more I glimpsed, in the exhibition hall where over 40 firms specializing in dialysis-related equipment had their displays, the extent of the huge medicoindustrial complex that has grown up around clinical nephrology. Nearly one billion dollars is currently being spent on the treatment of chronic uremia, mainly by the federal government. The phenomenal development of the technology of dialysis is both a cause and a result.

Most of the papers at the ASN meeting were concerned with the clinical or biologic aspects of renal disease, but at other gatherings of nephrologists, it is the technology that holds the stage. *It may be "half-way" technology, and it certainly is expensive, but without all those gadgets, we would still be back in the pre-1960 era, before nephrology became an important specialty and before it had anything to offer in the way of therapy.* The technology improves yearly.[13]

During the next eight years the "self-proliferating giant" along with the "expensive gadgets" would be examined closely and not always with such unquestioned confidence in clinical judgment.

Future accounts of clinical success in ESRD would take a very different, more guarded, form.

Clinical Statistics—The Picture of Effectiveness?

The quantitative picture of ESRD is a critically important part of the development of clinical theory. I do not mean this just in the sense of establishing an increasingly reliable and valid knowledge base for clinical applications, although this is obviously important. Given the highly uncertain nature of ESRD therapeutics, an image of clinical coherence seems a major part of the legitimation strategy for this new practice. In a very real way, clinical practice in ESRD has been left with a number of problems inherited from the limitation of a practice wholly based on high technology. There must be a framework to quantify the residual clinical uncertainty.

In a 1978 issue of *Clinical Nephrology* entirely devoted to a symposium entitled "Advances in Dialysis," this uncertainty is described: "At the same time too little is as yet known about the basic pathogenetic mechanisms of most kidney diseases, and large gaps which thwart their rational and curative treatment, or their prevention, still exist in our knowledge."[14] How is this type of ambiguity usually resolved within clinical theory? Often the randomized clinical trial (RCT) is used to establish the efficacy of a treatment approach. One might expect an RCT to be used to establish some baseline for clinical comparisons of outcomes in ESRD. There have been no major RCTs comparing modalities conducted on a representative sample of the Medicare-funded ESRD population. This is not surprising as RTCs are seldom used for emerging life-extending technologies, and in ESRD this pattern continues to be followed. The laissez faire nature of clinical theory in ESRD partially accounts for the lack of a major RCT. Some specific barriers include:

1. The strong association of renal physicians with a particular modality. Most nephrologists advocate one particular approach to treatment—hemodialysis, peritoneal, transplantation, etc.—as "optimal."
2. Increasing federal pressure generated by the Medicare ESRD treatment program. This has heightened awareness of effectiveness and efficiency in clinical practice and tends to make nephrologists "dig in" in defense of their favored modality.

3. The split of nephrologists into advocates or opponents of for-profit dialysis. This cleavage decreased the likelihood of a broadly based RCT because patient care and financial data are not freely shared between the hospital-based nonprofits and the free-standing proprietary treatment units.
4. The difficulty of a direct comparison and randomization. Given the nature of transplantation, patients would rarely be indifferent to the choice of dialysis versus renal transplantations, for example.

An RCT would, however, be unlikely to resolve the issue of uncertainty. The history of the major clinical trials in the United States indicates that the RCT is not the *deus ex machina* of truth for the assessment of complex medical technologies. Instead, the results of an RCT typically raise the level of ambiguity. This is because, as Marks argues,

what appear to be technical disputes concerning the design and analysis of this trial are in fact disputes about the standards by which evidence is to be judged, the weights to be accorded different kinds of evidence, and about the relevance of evidence from RCTs to resolving clinical disputes. I will also suggest that cognitive debates about the value of particular kinds of evidence are at the same time political debates about the value of different kinds of expertise, and that such debates are unlikely to be resolved solely by future improvements in the techniques of designing and analyzing RCTs.[15]

Critical Issues in Clinical Theory

Who gets renal failure? What causes ESRD? How do you treat it? What are the chances for long-term survival? Is there a serious decrease in the quality of life for surviving patients? These are the major questions confronting the clinical account of ESRD. Certain of these questions are embraced warmly within the clinical framework and others are shunned. Much of the controversy and most of the major clinical studies focus in three areas: (1) survival, (2) comparison of different treatment modalities, and—to a lesser extent—(3) rehabilitation of the ESRD patient. There is, of course, an extensive literature on the technical aspects of dialysis and transplantation involving immunological, physiological, bioengineering, and experimental studies on the pathogenesis of kidney failure among other areas. This is directed toward the nephrology community itself and is part of the infrastructure of professional activity most explicitly labeled "scientific." Like any other specialty in American medicine, this basic and applied clinical research is highly regarded as the bedrock of modern medical science and as forming a basis for future breakthroughs in clinical practice. My focus is, however, on a different category of clinical studies, those more directly related to the assessment of clinical practice and grounded in the more pragmatic problems of patient care. Also, my concern is with those issues more directly at the cutting edge of the clinical theory/effective therapy/ public assessment debates.

Who Gets Renal Failure?

Table 1 presents the changes in the composition of the patients receiving dialysis from 1967 to 1978. Clearly, the removal of cost barriers in 1972 had an important effect on the resulting social class of dialysis patients. In 1978 there were higher percentages of blacks, women, and persons fifty-five or older in the treated population. Obviously, clinical decisions regarding the treatable population were highly responsive to the availability of payment. Conversely, during the period of strictly limited funding for ESRD treatment, criteria for acceptable patients were much more narrow; the statistically ideal candidate from the 1967 profile would be a white male, college educated, less than forty years old, married, and employed. In sum, these shifts in the composition of the treated dialysis population reflect in part the social, economic, and political influence on clinical decision making among nephrologists and cautions against using the treated population as an unbiased proxy for true incidence or need.

The question of the incidence of ESRD (the rate of new cases of ESRD in the population) is barely addressed in the clinical literature. There are very few epidemiologically oriented studies available, and those studies range widely in their estimates from 60 per million to 200 per million.[16] Table 2 shows the best current (1984) estimates of the incidence of ESRD as reflected in the number of patients treated under the Medicare ESRD program from 1978 to 1980. As one would expect, the incidence of ESRD increases with age; this also follows the general patterns of chronic disease. The increased rate of ESRD among males compared with females (about 20 per million higher) is

Table 1
The Hemodialysis Patient Population in 1967 and 1978

Social and Demographic Characteristics	1967 (%)	1978 (%)	
Sex			
Male	75.0	49.2	
Female	25.0	50.8	
Race			
White	91.0	63.7	
Black	7.0	34.9	
Other	2.0	1.4	
Education			
Junior high school or less	10.0	28.7	
Some high school	17.0	17.2	
High school graduate	27.0	28.4	
Some college	20.0	18.2	
College graduate	12.0	5.7	
Postgraduate school	13.0	1.8	
Unknown	1.0	0.0	
Age			
Under 25	8.0	3.4	
25–34	24.0	10.0	
35–44	32.0	14.6	
45–54	27.0	25.8	
55 and over	7.0	45.7	
Unknown	2.0	0.5	
Marital status			
Single	16.0	13.0	
Married	79.0	61.8	
Separated		6.3	
Divorced	5.0	7.4	} 25.2
Widowed		11.5	
Employment status			
Employed	41.7	18.4	
Unemployed	38.3	17.7	
Disabled		53.6	
Student	13.2	Not coded	} 63.8
Retired		10.2	
Other	0.0	0.1	
Unknown	6.8	0.0	

Source: R. W. Evans, C. R. Blagg, and F. A. Bryan, "Implications for Health Care Policy: A Social and Demographic Profile of Hemodialysis Patients in the United States," *Journal of the American Medical Association* 245, no. 5 (1981): 487.

Table 2
Medicare ESRD Program Incidence Rates per
Million Population, by Age, Sex,
and Race, 1978–80

Social and Demographic Characteristics	1978	1979	1980	% Change, 1978–80
Total	71	78	82	15
Age				
0–14 years	6	6	7	17
15–24 years	26	26	24	−8
25–34 years	53	54	58	9
35–44 years	85	84	86	1
45–54 years	120	135	136	13
55–64 years	173	193	204	18
65–74 years	208	230	241	16
75 years and over	96	134	153	59
Sex				
Male	82	90	95	16
Female	61	67	70	15
Race				
White	59	63	67	15
Black	159	184	185	16
All other	118	131	140	19

Source: P. W. Eggers, R. Connerton, and M. McMullan, "The Medicare Experience with End-Stage Renal Disease: Trends in Incidence, Prevalence, and Survival," *Health Care Financing Review* 5, no. 3 (1984): 72.

an interesting finding, probably related to the increased rate of hypertension in males.

A major problem for clinical theory is the extremely high incidence of ESRD in blacks compared with whites, nearly three times greater in 1977. Although a number of studies have discussed this issue, there are few detailed assessments of this problem. Most clinicians consider this to be related to the increased incidence of hypertension among blacks, but even this is somewhat controversial and may involve the particular type of hypertension among blacks. Whatever the specific cause, the effect of this very high relative risk in blacks is a disproportional percentage of blacks among the population of treated ESRD patients (34.9 percent). (Certain urban-based ESRD treatment facilities have very large percentages of black patients, reaching 60 percent in some cases.)

This makes ESRD another of the end stages of disease that reflect the increased health risk for black populations. Within clinical theory the "problem of the black ESRD patient" represents a highly uncertain issue; some studies report that blacks are much more difficult to treat.[17] Other studies report that they are no more difficult to treat.[18] We will consider this issue again in the later chapters that are concerned with the relative complexity of patient care between hospitals and profit-making facilities.

What Causes ESRD?

Progressive chronic renal failure has many possible etiologies, including immunological abnormalities, infections, reactions to drugs, congenital abnormalities, vascular disorders, neoplasia, and trauma.[19] Renal failure may result from a specific disease of the kidney (renal related) or can also result from the effects of a systematic disease such as diabetes or hypertension. Because the first symptoms of renal failure occur very late in the course of the disease, it is usually difficult to assess the primary cause.

Available reports on the distribution of identifiable conditions that lead to kidney failure are generally inadequate in terms of the data used and also vary extensively in their findings. The sad state of epidemiological studies in ESRD reflects the allocation of research funds in the renal area—few resources have been spent on studies related to causes of kidney failure and possible approaches to prevention. The reason why prevention is not an area of active research is often stated as a self-fulfilling prophesy: "Dramatic advances in the prevention (or treatment) of ESRD do not seem imminent."[20] As a result, little research in prevention is conducted.

It is interesting to look at the distribution of primary diseases leading to ESRD. Table 3 presents data from the Medicare program. Almost 10 percent of the primary causes of chronic renal failure are unknown. Nearly 45 percent seem to result from systemic diseases

Table 3

Primary Diagnosis for Newly Entitled ESRD Persons, 1973–80

Diagnosis	1973 and Prior	1974	1975	1976	1977	1978	1979	1980
Number of persons	13,320	6,553	6,805	6,245	7,226	7,505	8,315	9,310
				Percent distribution				
All causes	100	100	100	100	100	100	100	100
Glomerulonephritis	36.4	29.2	27.1	24.7	23.5	21.7	21.0	19.7
Primary hypertensive disease	13.2	13.9	15.0	15.8	20.4	22.2	22.1	23.4
Diabetic nephropathy	7.0	11.9	12.2	14.0	15.8	18.0	18.7	21.8
Polycystic kidney disease	8.7	7.5	6.5	7.0	6.7	6.4	6.1	5.9
Collagen vascular disease	1.5	2.0	1.8	1.8	1.3	1.7	1.4	1.4
Interstitial nephritis, hereditary	1.5	1.4	1.0	1.6	1.2	.7	1.0	1.0
Interstitial nephritis, other	12.5	10.4	10.0	9.4	7.2	6.6	6.7	6.4
Analgesic abuse nephropathy	*	.1	*	.2	1.0	1.0	1.2	1.1
Obstructive uropathy, acquired	.3	.2	.1	.4	2.2	2.5	2.5	2.4
Obstructive uropathy, congenital	.1	.1	.1	.5	1.5	1.3	1.5	1.1
Amyloidosis	*	*	*	.1	.5	.6	.4	.5
Multiple myeloma	.1	*	.1	.1	.8	1.0	1.0	1.0
Gouty nephropathy	*	*	*	*	.3	.3	.3	.5
Other, unspecified	9.4	12.5	13.3	12.1	7.8	6.5	6.1	5.0
Etiology unknown	9.0	11.0	12.8	12.4	9.6	9.5	10.1	8.8

*Less than .1 percent.

Source: P. W. Eggers, R. Connerton, and M. McMullan, "The Medicare Experience with End-Stage Renal Disease: Trends in Incidence, Prevalence, and Survival," *Health Care Financing Review* 5, no. 3 (1984): 76.

(hypertension and diabetes), not from primary kidney disease. Poly-cystic kidney disease is a congenital condition. Interstitial nephritis is often caused by excessive exposure to analgesics (aspirin or phen-acetin), and chronic glomerulonephritis is the broad diagnosis most often found in patient records.

The opportunity for prevention, given the profile of causes, does not seem so grim as most studies suggest. Over 20 percent of ESRD results from hypertension, a condition that if detected early can be controlled, and the serious effects of the disease can be prevented. The association between interstitial nephritis and analgesics suggests another possible area for prevention. Finally, given the readily ac-knowledged deficiency in the federal data base and the difficulty of abstracting diagnostic information from medical records, some of the 10 percent of "unknowns" might also fall into categories where the condition may have been preventable, such as exposure to nephro-toxins (lead, pesticides) or toxics-related kidney damage. The fact that no detailed epidemiologic studies have been conducted to in-vestigate the reasonableness of a preventive strategy is unfortunate. Given the public and professional pressure on nephrology to present a clinical picture of technical success, such an absence of preventive studies is understandable. Prevention, then, has been effectively excluded from mainstream clinical theory in ESRD.

How Do You Treat It?

Perhaps the most active issue in ESRD clinical theory is the location and modality of treatments. In its simplest form the problem presents itself this way: There are two major forms of treatment, dialysis and transplantation. The treatment of ESRD in the United States is, essentially, a dialysis program. Over 80 percent of patients in the Medicare ESRD program are on some form of dialysis. Despite the inherent appeal of transplantation as a "cure" and the apparent improvement in the technology of transplantation (discussed below), this will remain the case for the foreseeable future. I will look at these two modalities in turn but, for the moment, not consider the issue of the relative costs of these treatment alternatives.

Dialysis can be provided either in hospital-based centers, in free-standing facilities (mostly for-profit), or at home. There are three types of dialysis. *Hemodialysis* and *intermittent peritoneal dialysis* may be performed either in a treatment center or at home. *Con-*

tinuous ambulatory peritoneal dialysis (CAPD) is usually done in the home and is a relatively new modality. Table 4 presents the distribution of patients across these modalities.

The most recent figures available (1983) show that 47 percent of the ESRD population was treated in hospital-based facilities, 39 percent in free-standing facilities, and 14 percent at home. The percentage of patients on home dialysis has dropped considerably since 1972 (40 percent), and there are wide-ranging estimates (25–40 percent by 1990) of the expected number of home patients in the future.[21] The best current estimate is that two-thirds of the home dialysis population uses CAPD. Physicians are largely the determining factor in the observed wide variation in the utilization of dialysis modalities among the states.[22] There are physician advocates for home dialysis,[23] for-profit free-standing dialysis,[24] hospital-based dialysis,[25] and CAPD.[26]

Much of the recent clinical literature is devoted to the question of "dueling modalities"—which form of dialysis is better (nephrologists

Table 4
Dialysis Treatment Modalities

Dialysis Type and Setting	*Number of Patients as of:*			
	12/31/80	*12/31/81*	*12/31/82*	*12/31/83*
In-unit staff-assisted hemodialysis	42,501	46,980	51,499	55,554
In-unit stall-assisted peritoneal dialysis	900	937	874	742
In-unit self-hemodialysis	770	1,030	1,060	1,475
In-unit self-peritoneal dialysis	11	7	11	3
Home hemodialysis	4,715	4,480	4,394	4,323
Home peritoneal dialysis	612	645	816	790
Continuous ambulatory peritoneal dialysis	2,334	4,333	6,523	8,532
Self-dialysis training:				
Hemodialysis	370	352	408	379
Peritoneal	45	26	19	33
CAPD	106	117	161	156
Total dialysis patients	52,364	58,924	65,765	71,987

Source: Health Care Financing Administration, "ESRD Program Highlights" (Washington, D.C., 1983).

use the term *optimal*). As we will see in Part II, "better" can be defined in many ways but most often will focus on relative costs, given some assertion of adequate survival and assessment of relative complications. Costs, however, are the ever-present specter in ESRD clinical theory, even in studies that are considered strictly biomedical such as studies of survival or of the complications of treatment. High-cost modalities are almost by definition on the defensive when they are evaluated; conversely, those modalities that promise lower costs can achieve quite a boost in the quest for therapeutic legitimation. This is because the requirements for clinical legitimation and bureaucratic legitimation intermingle in such a way that strictly clinical assessments of effectiveness seem necessary, but are not sufficient.

What Are the Chances for Long-term Survival?

If there is a tenet that forms the bedrock of clinical theory in ESRD (or biomedical science in general), it is the value of increased survival. The ability of a treatment to significantly extend a patient's life where no treatment would surely result in immediate death is almost in itself an operational standard for clinical effectiveness. "Dialysis or death" is a powerful symbolic contrast that invokes deeply rooted feelings of fear, mortality, and an ethical imperative. If a technology extends life, use it!

Survival, then, is the root of clinical theory in ESRD, and many of the important studies and reports of the clinical construction of this disease build upon this foundation. A close examination of these data reveals important controversies and ambiguities that highlight the patterns of uncertainty in the clinical construction of kidney failure.

Artificial or Transplanted Organs: Who Shall Live Longer?

As of December 31, 1983, the Health Care Financing Administration (HCFA) reported that there were 78,099 patients receiving treatment under the ESRD program. About 80 percent of these patients were receiving dialysis; only 20 percent were living with a functioning transplanted kidney. The questions of the outcome and effectiveness of dialysis versus transplantation is at the center of the survival issue. A large number of studies have attempted to analyze the relative effectiveness of the major modalities. As far as overall survival rates can be measured for the ESRD patients who are part of the federal program, the survival rates for both dialysis and transplantation have remained stable from 1977 to 1980; for all forms of dialysis, slightly over 80 percent of patients survive one year and roughly 56 percent survive three years. The survival rates for transplantation depend on whether the transplanted kidney comes from an unrelated donor (cadaver donor or CD) or a related donor (living related donor or LRD). In the case of CD about 86 percent of patients survive one year and approximately 78 percent survive three years. The corresponding figures for LRD transplants are 95 percent one-year and 91 percent three-year survival rates.[27] Table 5 presents a summary of survival rates related to a number of factors.

On the face of it, these data indicate that transplantation offers better survival rates and, therefore, the most effective method of treatment. Advocates of transplantation have used these survival figures and the rather loosely based notion that transplantation costs less than dialysis to recommend a greatly increased effort in transplantation. Carolyne K. Davis, former administrator of HCFA, cited the following "evidence" at a congressional hearing on organ transplantation: "a group of transplant patients would cost the Medicare program less than a group of dialysis patients after a four-year period."[28] Dr. Davis also contended that patients with functioning transplants are more likely to be employed and to have a lower level of physical impairment.

The case for transplantation would seem to be overwhelming: longer survival, better rehabilitation, and lower costs. Much of the current research literature in ESRD considers transplantation to be the wave of the future, a confidence based on the early success of a new immunosuppressant drug, cyclosporine, which protects against the rejection of the kidney transplant. The only problem is getting enough kidneys to transplant (*harvesting kidneys* is the pastoral terminology applied to this problem). As with most of the presentations of unambiguous success within the clinical construction, there is more uncertainty about transplantation than is immediately apparent.

Table 6 presents the survival rates of the *transplanted kidney* (graft-retention rate) according to the same characters examined in the patient survival rates in Table 5. This picture tells a somewhat different story and addresses a more specific aspect of effectiveness of transplantation: how long does the transplanted kidney work?

In the case of CD transplantation, one-year survival rates are approximately 56 percent and three-year survival rates only about 45 percent. The figures are better for LRD transplants: 75 percent and 67 percent for the one-year and three-year survival rates. These data indicate that *over 50 percent of CD transplants and 33 percent of LRD transplants fail after only three years*. Although the patient has a very high probability of surviving this interval and returning to dialysis, the kidney does not have so unambiguous a record of success. A recent study that adjusted for the effects of age and morbidity at the start of treatment found that there was no difference in survival between dialysis and CD transplantation and strongly suggested that this form of transplantation is not the nearly universal treatment of choice that advocates often suggest.[29] Also, survival is much poorer for subsequent transplants after an initial transplant fails.

To dull the veneer of success a bit further, over 70 percent of the kidneys transplanted in this country are obtained from cadavers,[30] which brings the overall kidney or graft-retention rate much closer to the CD figures than to the LRD rates. Finally, the performance of organizations that procure cadaver kidneys for transplantation are mixed, at best. Public attitudes about organ donation are not generally supportive and "marketing" attempts to encourage altruism must enter a complex web of family relations and attitudes concerning death.[31] The issues go far beyond the reach of simply improving public relations efforts.

Generic Considerations on ESRD Survival—Social and Clinical Factors

Three general dimensions are important components of the survival issue. First are the social and demographic characteristics of the patient. These include factors such as age, race, and income. Second is the clinical condition of the patient, which includes such things as type and extent of complicating conditions and the biological nature of the disease. And the third domain involves medical care factors, the modality used to treat a patient and the specific location of that treatment (hospital, home, or free-standing facility).

Table 7 presents a comparison of a number of studies of patients' survival on various types of dialysis. There is sufficient variability between different modes of dialysis (CAPD and hemodialysis) to raise a number of issues too detailed for a full discussion here but

Table 5
Survival Rates for Patients Receiving Dialysis or Undergoing
Transplantation, According to Various Demographic and Clinical
Characteristics*

Social and Demographic Characteristics	*Dialysis*		
	Survival to 1 Year (%)	*Survival to 3 Years (%)*	*No. of Cases*
Total	81 ± 0.2	56 ± 0.3	65,270
Sex			
Male	81 ± 0.3	55 ± 0.4	36,600
Female	82 ± 0.4	58 ± 0.4	28,581
Total			65,181
Race			
Black	85 ± 0.3	62 ± 0.5	17,194
White	80 ± 0.2	54 ± 0.3	43,990
Total			61,184
Age (yrs.)			
≤10	90 ± 2	82 ± 3	601
11–20	95 ± 0.5	88 ± 2	2,620
21–30	91 ± 0.5	78 ± 1	6,240
31–40	89 ± 0.5	71 ± 1	7,883
41–50	88 ± 0.4	68 ± 0.7	9,995
>50	77 ± 0.2	48 ± 0.3	35,911
Total			63,250
Primary disease			
Primary hypertension	82 ± 0.5	56 ± 1	7,049
Glomerulonephritis	91 ± 0.5	69 ± 1	6,538
Diabetic nephropathy	75 ± 1	39 ± 1	5,856
Polycystic kidneys	95 ± 1	78 ± 2	1,973

*The discrepancies in the totals are the result of exclusion of cases with missing data. In addition, results for the small, heterogeneous group of persons who were neither black nor white are not shown. The primary disease was identified in only about half of all cases, and only the major diseases are listed.

The plus-or-minus values are standard errors.

	Transplantation				
Unrelated Donor			Related Donor		
Survival to 1 Year (%)	Survival to 3 Years (%)	No. of Cases	Survival to 1 Year (%)	Survival to 3 Years (%)	No. of Cases
86 ± 0.4	78 ± 0.5	7,595	95 ± 0.4	91 ± 0.6	3,491
86 ± 0.6	77 ± 1	4,818	95 ± 0.5	90 ± 1	2,079
86 ± 1	78 ± 1	2,777	94 ± 0.6	91 ± 1	1,410
		7,595			3,489
86 ± 1	78 ± 1	1,625	93 ± 1	87 ± 2	364
86 ± 0.5	77 ± 1	5,588	95 ± 0.4	91 ± 1	2,905
		7,213			3,269
89 ± 3	80 ± 3	155	93 ± 2	89 ± 3	150
92 ± 1	87 ± 1	844	97 ± 1	95 ± 1	662
92 ± 1	87 ± 1	1,792	97 ± 1	95 ± 1	1180
85 ± 1	78 ± 1	2,016	93 ± 1	89 ± 1	798
81 ± 1	70 ± 1	1,737	91 ± 1	82 ± 2	490
79 ± 1	68 ± 2	1,051	88 ± 2	81 ± 3	208
		7,595			3,488
85 ± 1	77 ± 2	593	93 ± 2	86 ± 3	159
87 ± 1	81 ± 1	1,760	97 ± 1	93 ± 1	811
79 ± 2	65 ± 2	518	89 ± 2	82 ± 3	268
81 ± 2	77 ± 3	293	91 ± 3	82 ± 4	75

Source: H. Krakauer, J. S. Grauman, M. R. McMullan, and C. C. Creede, "The Recent U.S. Experience in the Treatment of End-Stage Renal Disease by Dialysis and Transplantation," *NEJM* 308, no. 26 (1983): 1560.

Table 6

Graft-Retention Rates According to Various Demographic and Clinical Characteristics*

Social and Demographic Characteristics	Unrelated-Donor Transplants			Related-Donor Transplants		
	Graft Retained 1 Year (%)	Graft Retained 3 Years (%)	No. of Cases	Graft Retained 1 Year (%)	Graft Retained 3 Years (%)	No. of Cases
Total	56 ± 1	45 ± 1	7,591	75 ± 1	67 ± 1	3,489
Sex						
Male	55 ± 1	44 ± 1	4,808	74 ± 1	65 ± 1	2,076
Female	58 ± 1	46 ± 1	2,776	78 ± 1	71 ± 1	1,409
Total			7,584			3,485
Race						
Black	50 ± 1	37 ± 1	1,624	64 ± 3	55 ± 3	364
White	58 ± 1	47 ± 1	5,578	79 ± 1	69 ± 1	2,901
Total			7,202			3,265

Age (yrs.)						
≤10	58 ± 4	46 ± 4	155	80 ± 3	71 ± 4	149
11–20	59 ± 2	46 ± 2	843	77 ± 2	68 ± 2	662
21–30	59 ± 1	48 ± 1	1,790	79 ± 1	72 ± 1	1,179
31–40	56 ± 1	44 ± 1	2,010	74 ± 2	66 ± 2	797
41–50	54 ± 1	42 ± 1	1,737	69 ± 2	58 ± 2	490
>50	52 ± 1	41 ± 1	1,049	68 ± 3	60 ± 3	207
Total			7,584			3,484
Primary disease						
Primary hypertension	52 ± 2	37 ± 2	593	65 ± 4	59 ± 4	159
Glomerulonephritis	55 ± 1	45 ± 1	1,758	76 ± 2	67 ± 2	809
Diabetic nephropathy	50 ± 2	39 ± 2	518	69 ± 3	59 ± 3	268
Polycystic kidneys	50 ± 3	43 ± 3	292	68 ± 5	60 ± 6	75

*The discrepancies in the totals are the result of exclusion of cases with missing data. In addition, results for the small, heterogeneous group of persons who were neither black nor white are not shown. The primary disease was identified in only about half of all cases, and only the major diseases are listed.

The plus-or-minus values are standard errors.

Source: H. Krakauer, J. S. Grauman, M. R. McMullan, and C. C. Creede, "The Recent U. S. Experience in the Treatment of End-Stage Renal Disease by Dialysis and Transplantation," *NEJM* 308, no. 26 (1983): 1561.

Table 7

Patient Survival on Continuous Ambulatory Peritoneal Dialysis (CAPD) and Hemodialysis (HD)

Population	Calendar Years	Dialysis Modality	N	Survival 1 year (%)	Comment
ESRD Program	1977–80	Predominantly HD	65,270	81	ESRD program enrollees beginning dialysis in 1977–80. The vast majority (98+%) of patients would have been on home or center HD in these years in an approximate ratio of 10:90.
Michigan Kidney Registry	1974–78	Center HD only	1,560	70.8	Actuarial survival curves calculated separately for patients on center HD only and all patients on center HD, including those subsequently transplanted or changed to another dialysis modality.
		All center HD	2,396	—	
EDTA Registry	1979–81	HD	—	84	Results in a low-risk "standard population" ages 20–60. Reference does not specify whether HD was home, center, or both.
		CAPD	—	78	
ESRD Program	1981	Home HD	109	91	ESRD program enrollees who began on dialysis between 1/1/81 and 3/31/81. The reference does not state whether survival rates are annualized or merely refer to survival in calendar year 1981 following enrollment.
		Center HD	2,929	86	
		CAPD	174	87	

Source: W. Stason and B. Barnes, *Effectiveness and Costs of Continuous Ambulatory Peritoneal Dialysis*, Office of Technology Assessment, Congress of the United States (Washington, D.C.: Government Printing Office, Sept. 1985), p. 27.

discussed at length elsewhere.[32] Looking back at Tables 5 and 6, we can summarize the factors that are particularly important for survival. Race is a complex determinant; blacks survive longer than whites on dialysis and on CD transplantation but demonstrate shorter survival on LRD transplantation. Further, graft-retention rates are far lower for blacks than for whites across all categories (see Table 6). There are no satisfactory explanations for these findings in the current literature. Certain physicians have suggested that, at least in the case of graft retention, this is not a racial factor but the influence of a particular treatment center. Centers that have a high success rate for functioning grafts just "happen" to have a predominantly white population of patient. Centers that are predominantly black "happen" to show the opposite trend. Such hypotheses represent the current state of the art in the clinical understanding of the effect of race on survival outcomes.

Other important risk factors affecting survival include diabetes (three-year survival on dialysis, only 39 percent) and age (three-year survival for patients over 65 on dialysis, 48 percent). These will be discussed more extensively in Part II of this book in connection with the general issue of case mix. At this point these data should be considered more as representations of the conventional wisdom of the clinical construction and less as empirically verifiable measurements.

Clinical Theory in ESRD: What's the Story?

In summary, these various components of the clinical construction of ESRD present a formal interpretation of highly variable and often poorly understood biological events. Clinical science assumes a role as a framework for objective discovery about disease processes. In the case of ESRD, this role is also very much a component of a framework of *justification* that is often acutely aware of and concerned with the public policy implications of "scientific" findings. The context of political legitimacy, which is the relative position of the clinical picture of ESRD compared with other (economic or bureaucratic) *competing* frames of problem definition, is a central, if unacknowledged, problem for nephrologists. Research findings that seem to fit the political and economic criteria for solution to the ESRD problem are supported, often without close or detailed review. CAPD, home dialysis, and even transplantation are heralded as cost effective without supporting evidence that examines so fundamental an issue as the case mix of patients selected for such modalities.

The clinical construction of ESRD is selectively considered in policy decisions and is also strongly influenced by the prevailing sentiment of cost-effectiveness assessments. Nephrologists or transplant surgeons adjust their science to the expected constraints of microeconomists in unconscious and often very subtle ways. As I will demonstrate further in later chapters, problems like the quality of life of patients and their families receive insufficient attention within the clinical construction. As a result, such experiential issues become even less central to the debate over federal policy for ESRD. In this way the social and cultural context of life-extending technologies like dialysis is stripped away. This pervasive, but elusive, intermingling of a clinical theory that clings to an abstract notion of objective medical science and an economic theory myopically focused on narrow cost parameters represents, unfortunately, a generic dilemma in health policy.

CHAPTER TWO

The Dynamics of the Experience of Illness

The preceding chapter has described the ways doctors create a clinical framework for ESRD. They reduce the wide-ranging biological and social complexity of the illness in an attempt to make the medical gaze internally consistent. By narrowing and fragmenting the scope of their clinical concern, doctors focus away from uncertainty and thus make the remaining problems appear more manageable. I questioned the extent to which a "managed" construction of the disease addresses the actual problems encountered in renal disease treatment. Such clinical construction of ESRD poorly articulates the problems of a patient's experience of illness. Moreover, clinical theory also provides an inadequate problem-solving context for the professionals who care for these patients.

In this chapter I will focus on the social dynamics of problem solving in ESRD treatment, on the effect that the *clinical way of knowing* has on the illness *experience*. Here, I define the illness experience as a social process in which the disease event is only one component. My methodological focus is directed toward a description and analysis of the multiple levels of meaning that constitute the dynamics of experience in ESRD. Data were collected during a two-year study of a hospital-based ESRD treatment program that offered all major forms of renal therapy (dialysis and transplantation). Participant observation was a major component of this study. I was a member of the hospital research staff and had access to all ESRD staff meetings, clinical conferences, and other day-to-day activities in the renal unit. Staff meetings and clinical conferences were tape recorded and abstracted to provide the excerpts included in this chapter. Interviews (semistructured) with the treatment staff and 50 patients were conducted, and detailed abstracts from the medical records of 150 ESRD patients were written during the eighteen-month period of this study.[1]

These data juxtapose diverse accounts, each of which provides a different approach to problem solving in ESRD care. The problems that are described generally represent the types usually encountered by patients with kidney failure.[2]

Organization of the Renal Unit

The renal unit was a part of a large teaching hospital in the Northeast, and most of the physicians held appointments in the affiliated medical school. The staff of thirty consisted of two full-time nephrologists, usually two renal residents who were in training, a nurse practitioner who coordinated patient care, nine nurses, five nursing assistants, and several renal technicians, who serviced the kidney machines. Part-time members of the staff included a dietician, a social worker, and a psychiatrist. This large number of staff members exemplifies the team concept in ESRD care, which is set up to provide specialized expertise in the various areas of treatment, from machine malfunctions to mental health.

The ways that the members of this team communicated with each other, conceptualized problems, and defined solutions were complex. The staff met twice each week to discuss important aspects of patient care. One meeting, involving only the nephrologists, other clinical "liaison" members (psychiatrist, residents), and the head nurse, was for the purpose of reviewing patients who had difficult problems during the previous week. These could range from a recent diagnosis of a tumor in a patient to a report by the head nurse that a patient's marriage was dissolving. Formal treatment plans might be proposed, although firm decisions were rarely reached during these meetings.

The second meeting of the week included the entire nursing staff, aides, the social worker, the dietician, and usually one of the nephrologists. Some of the information (but not all) from the first meeting was considered, although this was more of a gripe session for the staff than it was a patient care conference. As one nurse reflected,

"You can say what you want to in those meetings, and they listen to you, but you have no authority." General staff sessions could become quite boisterous, particularly so when a discussion of patients' home life ensued—in effect, a gossip session. Some members of the staff felt that too much discussion of intimate details of a patient's life took place:

> Why should all of the aspects of a patient's sex life be dragged out for the whole staff? What does the dietician need to know about a patient's sex life? It violates the confidentiality between the patient and the psychiatrist. I think there is too much discussion in those areas.

Staff members often disagreed about the best approach to a patient's problems. The head nurse, who had been with the program from its beginning, was a particularly assertive person. Many of the nurses complained in private that they had little input into decisions—what the head nurse says, goes. The physicians, for the most part, were less attuned to internal staff dynamics, as their interaction with the lower-level staff members was spotty and limited. As one nurse commented:

> Well there's a Monday morning meeting where only the doctors and the head nurse and the clinical specialists attend. The staff nurses are out in the trenches somewhere and unless you ask what happened at the meeting, no one tells you. Unless you see it written down somewhere. So it's kind of like a secret meeting.
>
> There's minutes—there's numbers—how many patients in, how many patients out, how many patients seen in the clinics. And they also bring up different patient problems. But it's not a group session for the entire unit. It's only for the ones that are in charge.

The problems of staff interaction are best understood in the context of particular patient care decisions, as I will discuss below.

As specialists in treating renal disease, the staff had difficult times in their relations with other departments in the hospital. The renal nurses were quick to point out that nurses in other hospital services, such as surgery or general medicine, were "scared to death" by dialysis and dialysis patients. They suggested that certain members of other hospital services questioned whether it is worthwhile to prolong kidney patients' lives. The following episode demonstrates how these opinions are formed.

A critically ill dialysis patient required surgery that was not related to his kidney disease. After a difficult operation the patient experienced serious complications in the recovery room. The surgical resident in charge of the recovery room called the chief nephrologist to tell him that, in his opinion, it would not be a proper use of the intensive care staff's time and energy to provide "heroic efforts" for this patient because, at best, he was "only going back to be on dialysis." This, of course, enraged the nephrologist, who immediately brought the matter to the attention of the hospital director and demanded that all life-sustaining efforts be made. The resident was overruled, treatment was continued, but the patient died anyway. The renal staff, in one of the weekly meetings, suggested that the surgical service was "incompetent." Given that the average ESRD patient over the course of treatment in this program has eight medical referrals outside the renal unit for serious problems, the misapprehensions of outsiders pose an ongoing problem for the staff of the renal unit.

Part of the problem of relating with other hospital departments in the medical center involved the perception of the clinical legitimacy of dialysis by other, more established specialties where there was less apparent uncertainty in treatment. As the medical director of the ESRD unit said to me:

> Well, for example, in academic institutions like ours, years ago dialysis was not considered a very scientific thing. It was not as sophisticated as working with a microscope and doing studies in basic science. However, we have been introducing the fact that dialysis is here and is taking care of hundreds of patients in this community. And each time there is a scientific meeting about renal disease, we present cases of dialysis problems. So I think that other members of the section that are not working directly in dialysis have begun to realize that dialysis is an important tool to treat a group of patients and has scientific aspects, room for improvement, and is part of modern-day medicine. I think that we are making progress, although I don't think as fast as I would like to.

Patients and the Illness Experience

Description of a few general characteristics of the patient population in this unit will provide a context for the case histories and staff excerpts that follow. Fewer than 10 percent of patients were employed full time, and 50 percent were not employed at all. The stress of dialysis is often too great to allow for the additional pressure of work. Moreover, many of these patients worked in occupations that involve manual work that demands a high degree of stamina. Most patients who did maintain full-time employment held professional-level jobs that were flexible enough to accommodate their ESRD treatment. The degree to which rehabilitation in ESRD is based on social class was also evident in this program; professional patients had a much more successful rehabilitation rate than those patients who had been blue-collar workers.

Most patients, with the exception of the few with successful transplantations, spent six hours a day, three days a week, attached to the dialysis machine, either at home or in the hospital. Some commuted, traveling 70 miles a round trip three times a week for their in-center dialysis. Home dialysis patients in this program lived as far as 250 miles away in another state. Many home-care patients came into the hospital only once every seven weeks.

Adjustment is difficult for ESRD patients. Although patients are told generally what to expect, no one is prepared for the dramatic changes that take place when treatment begins. For example, one man, who knew for ten years that his kidneys would eventually fail, was still severely jolted when the time to begin dialysis arrived. (He also lost his job when the treatments began.) "When we both [he and his wife] found out I was going on the kidney machine, we sat down at the table and cried like a couple of kids—What're we going to do? Who's going to take care of the family?" He went on to describe his initial peritoneal dialysis, the treatment usually given first because hemodialysis requires a prior surgical procedure:

It was a *humiliating* experience that I'll never *forget*. I'll never forget the first day. I seen that guy sticking those needles in me . . . it was a welcome to finally get on hemodialysis . . . welcome to my mind to think that I didn't have to go through this humiliation . . . of somebody sticking this sword into my stomach. I couldn't believe I had gone from a state of a guy who could take care of himself. . . . Here you've shrunk to a position that if you don't get this thing stuck in you . . . (he trails off).

Once renal dialysis has begun and the initial adjustment to this therapy has passed, the patient continues to be under a great deal of stress. Between dialysis treatments, excess fluids build up and may cause the patient to be bloated. (Dialysis patients do not urinate.) As the level of metabolites and waste products slowly rises, many patients feel dizzy and often have reported that "their thinking gets fuzzy." Diet becomes a regular battle, as the types of food dialysis patients can eat is limited; no foods with high potassium or salt content are allowed (most fruits, tomatoes). Total fluid intake must be carefully monitored—usually restricted to one cup per day. Diet is an area around which there is much patient-staff conflict. Many of the nurses consider that a "successful" dialysis patient is one who comes in for treatment no more than three pounds overweight. If the patient is sufficiently over the prescribed weight, the nurse has to "take off" the excess fluid by increasing the pressure of the blood flow through the dialysis machine. This is a difficult procedure, as it is quite painful, and it also requires extra work for the nursing staff.

For most ESRD patients, the nurses and technicians are their most important contacts. The nephrologist sees most patients infrequently. The relationships between the nurses and the patients are extremely important to the care process because of the extensive contact between them. The nurses know the families of most patients.

There is considerable stress within the families of ESRD patients. The staff attempts to help the families cope with the pressures, often suggesting group therapy. A number of dialysis patients in this unit went through divorces, many shortly after the treatment began. Staff members, however, believed that it was not the stress of dialysis per se that caused the trouble. As the chief nephrologist explained:

> We have to realize that when we get patients who have renal disease and need dialysis, we are getting a human being who has had many other problems in the past. Couples who are getting a divorce are couples who have had problems for years and kidney disease and dialysis is *just another event*.

The notion that ESRD constitutes "just another event" is one that the nephrologist can hold only because of the distance between himself and the experience of the patient. The nurses are more attuned to the social and emotional problems generated by ESRD and tend to get very involved in those aspects of the patients' lives. Their involvement, however, is influenced by their role as clinicians, which carries with it most of the assumptions of clinical theory. The line between becoming humanistically involved in the social aspects of a patient's experience and extending clinical social control is a fine one. Sometimes the staff's best-intentioned efforts result ultimately in actions that fall into the latter category. In cases where staff members became concerned about a patient's marital conflicts, they often forced the couple to accept psychiatric treatment. There were instances in which the head nurse called a patient's wife to tell her that she did not think the wife was sufficiently supportive. Social control in this chronic disease treatment setting, then, is an important issue. The subtle coercion that is implicit in the provider-patient relationship is often sufficient to endow the provider with considerable control.

In ESRD treatment, moreover, the staff does have recourse to an ultimate power in managing patients' behavior—they have control over life and death. This power is sometimes exercised, as the following incident demonstrates.

The Threat to Deny Dialysis

One problem discussed repeatedly during staff meetings was the possibility that some patients had been exposed to hepatitis. Hepatitis outbreaks are one of the complications that a dialysis staff fears most. Because of the daily exposure of the nurses to blood, hepatitis infections can spread rapidly among both patients and staff. Younger, female nurses are particularly fearful of hepatitis because of its deleterious effect on pregnancy outcome. Dialysis units are categorized as either "clean" or "dirty"—depending on whether they treat patients with hepatitis or do not. This hospital is a "clean" unit, which partially explains the extent of the staff's anxiety.

The patient being discussed was a twenty-eight-year-old unemployed former heroin addict who was on chronic renal dialysis at a satellite facility at another hospital in the state. The staff believed that in his last visit to the central unit he had exposed other patients to hepatitis. The "problem" was to substantiate this diagnosis by bringing the patient in for tests. The doctor said, "I think that we should bring him to the hospital. We can control him here. I also want to run a biopsy on him." A biopsy is a painful diagnostic procedure. All the staff seemed to agree that this would be a good way to get the patient to come in. They also agreed that the biopsy really would not tell them anything. A few days passed, and the patient refused to come in. The doctor declared, "I think what we should do is to tell him that if he wants us to continue to sponsor his dialysis, he'd better come in for this biopsy or we will *deny* him dialysis." A week went by, and the patient still refused to come in.

> *Nurse*: Something really has to be done about this. We've tried to get him in. I don't think that he'll come in. We have to call the nurse at the unit and tell her *not* to dialyze him until he comes in to us.
>
> *Doctor*: Well, I'll back you up on this.
>
> *Resident*: This guy is really a problem, he's an unreliable patient.
>
> *Nurse*: Yes, I get bad vibes from this patient.
>
> *Nurse*: Well, when we get him up here, we will straighten him up.

Under this threat, the patient came in. He was not a hepatitis carrier, as subsequent tests discovered. Because this man had been previously labeled a "difficult patient," the staff felt justified in their actions. The fact that he had been a heroin addict also legitimated their course of action.

The Iatrogenics of Authority Maintenance

Most members of the treatment staff were threatened when a patient questioned their clinical expertise. Dialysis patients come to know a great deal about the mechanics of the artificial kidney and, in many cases, can dialyze themselves better than the nurses can. Certain patients begin to feel very confident and consider themselves as knowledgeable about their illness as the clinical staff. A condescending phrase that often cropped up in the medical record notes and also in the staff meetings was "the patient attempts to use medical terms when describing his condition." A variant of this was another descriptor usually applied to the "problem" patient: "She has her *own* ideas about things!" What these labels seem to imply is that patients overstepped the "understood" bounds of acceptable behavior when they attempted to reason for themselves, rather than passively accepting the staff's pronouncements on their medical condition. The following example illustrates the dynamics when a patient struggled to understand his illness in his own terms but was opposed by the treatment staff, who withheld information in order to maintain control.

Mr. O. was a fifty-five-year-old white man who had been married for thirty-two years. He had bought a camper-trailer in which he planned to install his dialysis machine and travel around the country. Mr. O. had been employed on a part-time basis as a supervisor in an engineering management firm, except when he had in-patient treatment. He was a knowledgeable and assertive individual who seemed to know what he wanted out of life.

Two years before our interview, Mr. O. had had some problems with the dialysis staff concerning the cause of severe symptoms he was experiencing. After the staff changed the company that supplied the dialysis solution, Mr. O. began to experience weakness, nausea, vomiting, and intestinal irritation whenever he would dialyze.

Then they changed supplies of the solution. *That* solution made me sick. I just went down hill for three months. It took me that long to find what was causing it. Then I lengthened the time between treatments to four days. I'd get to feeling pretty good, then I'd have a treatment and get sick again. I also, with more or less of the doctor's consent, put 3 percent water in the solution, to make it weaker. This helped because I figured whatever was doing this to me wouldn't be as strong. It took me *until a year and a half* to convince the doctors that it was the solution. The doctors had said that there was no way that they could find out if the solution was the cause. Up until it had been one year, they said that it *couldn't* be caused by the solution. That was their answer. Every time I would see them [the doctor] I would tell them that the solution was still making me sick. I got no *action*. Finally, after a year and a month they did change it.

While Mr. O. was attempting to convince the doctors that his solution was the source of his problems, his case was discussed in the Monday staff meetings.

Doctor: This man displays bizarre behavior. I just don't understand him. He's angry at the staff because he feels that he's been "mismanaged." I think that his mentation is inappropriate.

Dietician: I don't like him. He has "fixed ideas."

Psychiatrist: I just don't understand. He used more reason in the past. They used to be a model couple. We used them as an example during the grand rounds.

Doctor: He even has "ideas" about his androgen therapy, claims the other one was better, more potent. Well, I think he should see a psychiatrist.

As a solution to this "problem" (they considered the problem to be Mr. O.'s behavior), the staff doctors decided to paste a different label on the same dialysis concentrate fluid and try to convince Mr. O. that they had made a real change. The staff, however, felt that he was too smart to be fooled by this tactic for very long. As Mr. O. related:

> Then they changed it, but it was still not good. This one made me sick—gave me fever blisters, sores in my nose, sores in my head, sores in my rectum. I was so weak, that in the last two years I couldn't travel, even around town. I couldn't take care of my car or the yard or do the other things I had done up to that time. I had a bladder cancer operation after that.

Mr. O. had complained to the staff for many months about the sores in his rectum, but to no avail. Finally this was brought up in a staff meeting.

Nurse: Now he's complaining about lesions in his bowels.

Doctor: Well, let's order a full G.I. and brain scan; if it's not somatic, then we'll send him to a psychiatrist.

He had developed a cancer in his bowel, although the treatment staff presented this as a problem "in his head." Even after this incident, the staff attempted to make another false change of the concentrate. As predicted, Mr. O. was difficult to fool:

> And they changed it after that, but the second changed solution, it bothered me too; and I ended up with an elbow swollen to 13½ inches. . . . I felt better, but tle sores and my elbow swelled, and I had a temperature of 104, so I went to the hospital and they told me. "You're not going home tonight." They didn't know what it was; couldn't draw any "cultures" from the elbow fluid. Between the fluid taps and the antibiotics, it got me pretty weak.

The continued problem presented by Mr. O. had begun to visibly upset certain staff members, particularly the head nurse.

Doctor: Now he's got a "swollen left elbow."

Dietician: This is a really difficult personality, he's got rigid ideas.

Nurse: He's crazy.

Doctor: He's going downhill. He just seems to have his own ideas about things.

For the staff, the "problem" with Mr. O. was that he was crazy. For Mr. O., the "problem" was otherwise:

It didn't bother anyone else. I mean there were thirty other guys on it. I was the only one complaining about it. Dr. Matthews said he never heard or read about anything like that. But they had no idea themselves. . . . Even though they say that a person who is their own doctor has a fool for a patient, I've been right. I study things out. I stretched out treatment, diluted the solution, lowered the pressure in the machine. That all helped. I tried all these things out. I had tried these things out. I didn't first jump into anything. I tried to find out the cause, but I just couldn't convince them. It was bad, frustrating. . . . I didn't ask if I could buy my own solution. I thought that if I bought my own stuff that they'd disown me. What I wanted . . . I figured that when I went over there I'd get some help at the clinic. Each time I expected help when I complained. The last time I talked to Dr. Matthews—I don't know if he knew it or just felt it, but I had made up my mind at that time, if he didn't give me help I would go to the top of the hospital, both to the surgical and social part. It had just gone on too long, you know. Then he said that he'd change it again for me.

By this time, after Mr. O. had developed two tumors and an "idiopathic" swollen elbow, the dialysis concentrate was *actually* changed. As Mr. O. told the story, "Then I switched to the Cobes solution and the elbow went down an inch and a half, right there during the treatment, and the pains went away. I've had no fever blisters, sores in my nose or head, or any feeling of it making me sick since." He went on to summarize the whole experience:

Only when Betty [the nurse-coordinator] came back did they do something about it. This is the problem with that hospital, nobody will *listen* to the patient. I felt that due to that I was sick a year more than I should have been; plus, it was the cause of all my trouble now. If you keep something unattended for a year and a half you're going to develop cancer or something. And I figure that's how I got cancer in my bowel. I had gotten hemorrhoids, sores, all since that solution. . . . 90 percent of the people would not listen to me, or they would try to make me like I was stupid and didn't know what I was talking about. This was the feeling they gave me because they were so blunt in saying it *isn't* the solution. And I mean from the nurses on down, with few exceptions. They felt loyalty to the doctor or something, but they gave me a rough time. I went over there for one treatment and I told the gal about it and she said that she couldn't change the solution like I did at home. And I says, "well, you can do one thing—at least keep the pressure low." Well, she looked at me and saw that I was a little overweight, so she put the pressure right up to the maximum. This made me real, real sick for about six weeks, this one treatment.

Months after this incident, Mr. O. was in the hospital again for metabolic treatments. He felt that these procedures were making him sicker and wanted to leave. The staff persisted in refusing to consider his ideas, even when they knew he might be correct.

Doctor: He wants to go home; says that the aluminum is poisoning his bones.

Resident: Can't we just slip him some [metabolic treatments]?

Dietician: Nope, he's too smart for that.

Nurse: Looks like he knows his body best.

Dietician: Please, don't anybody show him that recent article about aluminum causing bone lesions in dialysis treatment.

For the most part, the dialysis staff appeared reluctant to accept a patient's judgment concerning a medical problem. In Mr. O.'s case, two years and many serious complications later, the staff still would not consider his conjectures as legitimate. This would appear to be related to the avoidance of uncertainty, described previously, that permeates the clinical theory of ESRD. So much is unknown that it becomes quite threatening when a patient is able to diagnose a symptom when the doctor cannot. In Mr. O.'s case, the staff's reluctance to accept the validity of his complaints generated an iatrogenic outcome.

The unmanageable nature of ESRD presents itself in many ways. In a sense the exceptions to the rules far outnumber the events that go by the books. Dialysis solutions are not supposed to cause cancer, but perhaps they do. ESRD is not supposed to cure itself, but, as the next case illustrates, even this sometimes occurs.

Mr. H. was a fifty-two-year-old unemployed former truck driver. His medical chart prominently noted that he was a former alcohol abuser. Mr. H. had also been labeled as a wife abuser, and the staff psychiatrist predicted that he would have a "difficult future course and will continually test the staff." The course of his renal disease was rapid; he arrived at the hospital's emergency room one evening and was immediately placed on dialysis.

A little over one year after his admission to the ESRD program, these unusual events transpired. Mr. H. was said to have developed "problems" since he went on home dialysis. Instead of following the prescribed three-times-a-week schedule, he had been dialyzing only two times a week. Mr. H. said that he "didn't feel he needed it," that "he felt fine," and, not only that, he told them that he had begun to make urine again. The doctors found this totally unbelievable and called him in to take a series of renal function tests. When the results of the tests became available, they discovered that his kidneys had begun to function again—the cells had regenerated. He had improved so much that he did not need dialysis. This news, however, presented the staff with a problem—they did not know what to do or how to handle this information.

Doctor: How do we explain this to him? I mean, how do we account for this?

Nurse: What do we do? Do we just tell him that he doesn't need to dialyze anymore—that he's cured?

Psychiatrist: I don't think that it's a good thing at all just to tell this man he's "cured," and just let him go. Anyway, how do you know the urine sample he sent in is *really* his urine? I think that we should keep him in somehow.

After some discussion, the decision was reached *not* to tell the patient that his kidneys were functioning well enough on their own. The doctor said to tell him that he was getting good enough dialysis that he only needed once-a-week treatment. The plan was to suggest to the patient that he and his wife join a couples' therapy group with the psychiatrists. In these sessions the psychiatrist would tell them about the recovery and help them deal with this change. Over a month passed before the patient was told that his kidneys were functioning and that he could stop the treatments.

Clinical Theory and Treatment Realities

Mr. H.'s case presented a conceptual jolt to the treatment staff, who could not accept the idea of a spontaneous cure. It threatened them, in a sense, because it provided another example of their lack of control over the course of illness events in their unit.

The avoidance of uncertainty that permeates the clinical theory of ESRD can be seen in many of the events and situations I observed.

The continual presence of a large number of "non-renal complications" in their patients dominated the problems of patient care for the clinical practitioners in ESRD. What clinical theory constructs as an external problem, then, becomes a core problem for the practitioners and patients involved in the dynamics of treatment. Most patients in this program had numerous chronic conditions, some that developed prior to renal failure and others subsequent to it. The staff spent most of its time attempting to manage these conditions. Many of these complications were simply not understood and were treated as anomalous events, even though they appeared quite frequently. As one renal physician commented, referring to the very high number of deaths in dialysis patients from congestive heart failure: "Quite a few of our patients have fluid on the heart—some drop dead and some don't. What can you do?"

When a patient was discovered to have a terminal "nonrenal" complication, the treatment staff was at a loss as to how to deal with it. Usually, the event was taken out of their hands by other specialists, which tended to reinforce their sense of a lack of control.

There seems to have been little in the training of these ESRD specialists that prepared them for treatment realities. The staff's expertise in dialysis at best prolonged patients' lives but did not cure them. The plethora of complications that the patients experienced was frustrating for the treatment staff and life-threatening for the patients. Both had a difficult time coping, as the following example indicates.

Complications, Referrals, and Death

Mr. N. was a fifty-six-year-old retired machine operator in a rubber plant. He experienced many difficulties in his ESRD treatment over the years. Less than one year after he began dialysis, a malfunction in the machine caused an air embolism to be introduced into his bloodstream. Mr. N. survived, but he never regained confidence in the dialysis procedure. During the next six months he attempted "suicide" three times, according to his medical record (although a careful review of his medical record indicates that it is unclear exactly what he had attempted to do).

Two years later his first cancer was discovered (a lung tumor). He recovered from cancer surgery only to have another tumor diagnosed after another two years. The staff physician reported this new finding in this way:

The tomograph showed that he had a bony tumor around the lung that really got the house staff excited. . . . I don't know why we should talk with N. concerning the tumor. He doesn't want to know anything. When we removed the first one, he asked, "Doc, am I alive and cleaned up?" I don't think he wants information, because he doesn't ask questions. If he's not curious, then it's not my responsibility to tell more than the patient seems to want to know.

The doctors decided not to tell Mr. N. because they felt that the tumor was inoperable and would probably grow slowly. They would tell him later. For the time being, they told Mr. N. that the tumor was benign. Mr. N., however, did not believe this and got very upset. He began to vomit frequently and said, "All this started with this tumor." The staff could find no "medical" reason for this vomiting. The doctor said, "I've worked him up *ad nauseam*. This vomiting cannot be medical. It has to be psychiatric."

Mr. N. continued to vomit and became weaker. He also became dejected and upset. The staff psychiatrist saw him and admitted him to the psychiatric ward with this diagnosis: "Mr. N. displays depressive affect and psychogenic vomiting that has become life threatening. This is probably a slow form of suicide."

During this psychiatric admission, Mr. N. was placed on a bland diet, which consisted only of eggs, milk, and macaroni. This was not necessary, but the psychiatric staff was, in effect, frightened by this ESRD patient. They mentioned in his medical record notes that he had "disrupted" the entire psychiatric service because they were not prepared to deal with "sick people." The nurse in charge of this service felt that Mr. N. was also "suicidal" and in his medical record described his suicidal behavior:

Patient had refused to eat selected food on his supper tray. Staff offered to call kitchen for replacement. Patient refused offer. Later in the evening he came to staff demanding his cupcakes. The bag, in fact, housed a boiled ham and cheese sandwich. It was not given to the patient and he became angry and grabbed a nurse to retrieve the bag of food. He was asked to be patient and wait until his clinician could be called and consulted with. He went in to the

TV room and grabbed an apple from a fellow patient. It was half eaten (skin and pulp) when staff saw him. He was restrained.

Patient is hungry—due to not eating proper diet. Possibly suicidal?

Staff offered patient snack after consulting nurse on dialysis unit and patient's clinician.

There was no reason Mr. N. could not have eaten this sandwich, as he had regulated his own diet for years and knew how to balance his food intake. The man, in fact, was starving. A few days later he decided to leave the psychiatric service "against medical advice"(AMA). This was reported to the staff by the team psychiatrist.

Nurse: This AMA, can he really do that?

Doctor: Mr. N. has decided to sign himself out AMA. I called the psychiatrist and he said that the patient is not improving—that it would take a couple of months.

Psychiatric resident: He's had no response with anti-depressants; next we'll try electroshock. He has this fixed delusional system around his vomiting.

[Nurses are appalled at young psychiatric resident's glib description of what electroshock entails: nine times a week—"zonking," "eyelids flutter," "a few convulsions," "some foaming at the mouth."]

Nurse: Do the psychiatrists really know what they are doing? They called him a "management problem"—too many dietary charts ["patient eating apple . . . *not* his own"].

Psychiatrist: He should be stable, but he's not allowing the staff to help him—the psychiatric staff is not used to *medical problems*.

Psychiatrist: I feel that he's suicidal, and I want to get an outside psychiatrist to commit him.

Mr. N. was not committed, however, because the psychiatric staff felt that they would not be able to convince legal authorities that the man was incompetent.

After this stressful experience with psychiatry, Mr. N. went home only to come down with acute pericarditis. By this time, the staff had become quite upset about him.

Doctor: Seems ready to go; he doesn't know about the pericarditis. I don't want to record this death as pericarditis.

Resident: This is a really unpleasant person that demands things of us which we have no control. . . . I don't like to see him; I want to visit him less and less.

Psychiatrist: You should send him back to psychiatry *now*.

Psychiatric resident: I think it's his libido; he's pretty depressed . . . not much there.

Nurse: I had a dream. I saw Mr. N. in a dream and I said "quit feeling so sorry for yourself!" And I gave him quite a kick in the butt and he said "OK, Mandy!"

Mr. N. died two weeks later.

In this case the clinical staff had difficulty accepting that they were powerless to help Mr. N. Instead of accepting the fact that he had cancer and that there was nothing that they could do, they chose not to tell him. When he became upset and incredulous, they labeled his problems "psychogenic" and sent him to psychiatry. The psychiatric service, not used to "sick people," was threatened by his disease and overreacted by almost starving him. The dialysis team, upset about the multiple problems that this patient developed, began to dispute among themselves as to what the problem was. In the end, their concern was that his death not be recorded as another negative survival statistic against the track record of the unit.

Understanding the Crisis of Experience

A blind sixty-year-old dialysis patient described very well the way a patient experiences the crisis of dialysis, as opposed to the way clinicians view such stress. Here he recounted his personal view of the natural history of his illness.

They finally came in and told me I had been selected—they were going to put me on dialysis and I would start dialysis within a day or so. I was happy, because it looked as though dialysis would be the answer to the problem I was facing—little did I know that dialysis wasn't. . . . I did very well in dialysis first two or three years—I was strong. . . . Dialysis was, at first, just a side issue. . . . It didn't affect my life . . . except it limits how much you can travel.

I don't know when dialysis began to become burdensome . . . not hardly while I was working . . . but it did change in nature after about four years . . . and I can tell you when it did really change psychologically—and that's when we went on three days instead of two. Up until about five years ago—twice a week—dialysis was not a problem for me, until I began to go on dialysis three days a week. . . . You feel better and that's the medical side of it, but the psychological side of it is that when you have to start going to dialysis every other day, the build-up psychologically is something I don't think they realize yet—I don't think they know what it means to the patient to have to dialyze every other day. I mean once upon a time, we had several days in between dialysis and there was this feeling of *being yourself*, of having control of your own life. But every-other-day dialysis really takes that away—and now I will find guys taking "mental health days" [unauthorized days off dialysis]—You have to. . . .

Doctors have never come to ask us how do we feel about three days on dialysis.

You're psychologically tired—and then when something happens on the machine—it got to the point where I broke down in tears on the machine and, I don't know why—I'm just whipped to death, and then in a day or so, I come out of the slump.

No one talks about the real problems they were having with their families, or the fact that they had to quit their job, because they could no longer perform them. There are a lot of problems amongst these patients that are left undug!

I've reached the point now, though, where I have deteriorated at a double rate. I've lived eight years on the machine, but it feels like 16–20 years have passed. What it does to the body, what it does to you—my resolve is not what it used to be . . . it may not be just dialysis—but it has taken its toll. You cannot eliminate it as a great do-er, a kind of destroyer at work—it keeps you alive, that's for sure, but at the same time it's doing that, it's . . . maybe it's that way . . . if you're going to live to be 72, and you're on dialysis, it would be my guess, my layman's guess, that dialysis would probably cut about eight years off your life. . . . It feels like you're wearing out faster.

I can see how I'm reacting to dialysis as compared to when I first went on. *Now*, when I come off dialysis, it takes me six hours to overcome the dialysis itself—there was once upon a time when I almost danced out of the hospital—now—I come out like a dish-rag—[it takes about six hours] to reintegrate—I just feel scattered.

If I were a 22-year-old man, with dialysis facing me . . . [laughs].

These excerpts reveal aspects of the dialysis patients' experience that are less known and perhaps inaccessible to clinical theory. Psychiatrists can listen to statements such as these but rarely step back and consider the complexity of feelings and conflicts, as these notes written by a psychiatrist on Mr. H.'s medical record indicate:

The patient appears severely depressed all the time. He always appears on dialysis as if he were ready to cry or die. He is hard to deal with because he has numerous complaints about which there is no help for him. He is, after all, going blind and on chronic dialysis. He is a demanding person and difficult to give psychological support to.

The patient struggles to understand the experience of uncertainty while the physician struggles to *exclude* uncertainty from experience.

Death in Dialysis—Contrasting Perspectives

When a patient did die while on dialysis, particularly one who was not expected to die, the staff viewed the problem as a challenge to their professional expertise. One nurse described what the staff called "machine deaths": "Hopefully, when somebody dies on the machine, it's been somebody who's been going downhill anyway. . . . Then it's a little easier. It's always easier to pin *it* on something else. It's a lot easier to say he had a heart attack than to say he just failed to thrive—it's a lot easier to deal with."

The head nurse also recognized the traumatic aspects for staff members when there was a death in the unit, but believed that the standard procedures attempted to meet the needs of surviving patients.

Generally, if it occurs during dialysis here, it's generally then a very traumatic situation with codes being called and all kinds of people rushing and this kind of thing. . . . There's no division curtains, for instance, so they witness the whole thing and it's been kind of hectic. I think one of the good aspects, if you can find something good about it, is that they've seen that everything's done that is possible to do. And so they know that if, for instance (and they all internalize it), "it could happen to me" they do know that everything's going to be done for them. But depending on how long they've known the particular person—and perhaps it's been somebody that they've been able to communicate with—it depends on what kind of reaction they have. We're very open with them. For instance, if somebody dies in a different area, we still share it with all the patients because they're going to know about it, and if we don't tell them, then they're gonna wonder—why did we keep it from them. And so we share it with them and talk about it. We frequently cry with them over it.

Mr. H., whose comments were presented at length previously, had this to say about the way the staff handled a death in the unit:
Another thing that's disturbed me, ever since I've been there, is dying patients—dying is mysterious enough—I've seen this often enough when someone died, right there, in the unit. But then I've also not been there, and someone died, and you wake up one day and say, "I haven't seen Joe around for awhile." And you say, "Listen, what happened to Joe Jones?" "Oh," they say, "he passed away three days ago."
And that's a hell of a thing to do. You just let him sort of fade away—don't you say?
I'd rather be told—I don't know why. . . . There's no mention—his name isn't said. . . . He just isn't there. . . . That's always disturbing to me.

CHAPTER THREE

Negotiation, Compromise, and Conflict
The Network of Survival

Trust totally in a life-giving machine, but bear the constant fear of dying. Hope for understanding and support from health care providers and loved ones, but be met often with frustration and guilt. Change your diet, give up your job, and adapt to a new physical appearance. Imagine yourself coping with all these challenges to your usual lifestyle, and you will begin to appreciate the experience of illness in ESRD.

On the other hand, envision teaching a life-saving treatment regimen to a reluctant patient or the constant sense that your best clinical efforts cannot control your patient's illness, and you will gain some understanding of the situation of health care providers who provide care for a chronic renal failure patient. Obviously, imagination alone cannot provide a clear conception of the experiential dynamics of ESRD. Rather, it must develop from an assessment of all of the forces affecting the life and care of the patient.

This chapter does not focus solely on patient management issues from a health care provider's vantage point. Nor is it merely an attempt to classify the patient's "psychopathological" symptoms. Rather, by critically analyzing the existing research literature on chronic illness (and ESRD in particular), we will examine what I call the "professional/objective" understanding of the dynamics of the ESRD illness experience. What construction of patients and clinical problems emerge from this framework? How do the assumptions of the "professional/objective" frame influence our wider public perceptions of ESRD and, ultimately, health policy? Through these and other questions, we can come to understand the sources of the tensions and conflicts we have seen in the previous chapter.

To conceptualize the social and experiential aspects of ESRD, think of a set of concentric circles. The societal forces (federal health policy or the dialysis industry) are represented by the outermost ring; the health care providers (treatment unit staff, psychiatrists), by the next ring; the patient's social support system (friends and family), by the circle within that; and the patient is the core. Conventionally, the flow of information and services goes toward the center; that is, clinical paradigms and treatments are *applied* to the patient. How can we explore the patient's own view of these psychosocial dynamics, given the dominance of these external forces?

The "Public" Problem of ESRD

In analyzing the "public" perspective, we must view chronic illness as a political process rather than simply as a form of individualized deviant behavior. As Gerson explains, the traditional functionalist, medical-sociological conception of illness, couched in such terms as *deviance, sick role, compliance/noncompliance*, precludes a complete understanding of the patient's plight at a systemic level: how illness operates within our political-social organization.[1] Given the historical shift in the focus of medical care from acute to chronic care and, likewise, the parallel shift from cure to long-term management, a conflict of interest between the physician and patient can arise: while the physician exerts control to manage both her work and the disease as best she can, simultaneously, the patient must manage his disease *and* the impact of the physician's management decisions on his quality of life. Catastrophic and chronic illnesses like ESRD involve sophisticated and complex medical technologies. Obviously, the medical personnel are knowledgeable in the use of such technologies and are highly competent in the technical aspects of treatment protocol. It is less well known that an extremely high level of sophistication is also demanded of the patient and his social support system. Because complete recovery from the illness is unlikely, the more realistic goals are long-term treatment and rehabilitation. The patient, the family, and the care providers, then, embark on a journey in which they interact closely over a (it is hoped) long treatment period. These relatively highly enmeshed patient, family, and provider interactions occurring over a long time (up to ten years) typify the illness experience of ESRD and are in sharp contrast to the more usual provider/patient interactions in acute care.

Much of the current literature that considers ESRD reduces the multifaceted human problems associated with kidney failures to issues such as efficiency of care, regulation of reimbursement, or the cost-benefit ratios of new approaches to treatment. Although this approach to problem definition is understandable, and perhaps unavoidable, it nevertheless supports a narrow and piecemeal approach—reducing costs here, raising ethical questions there. This form of inquiry is consistent with the conventional approach to medical care analysis but obscures the unusual dynamics of ESRD treatment that, if comprehensively considered, can broaden our understanding of the problem of chronic illness.

A misinterpretation of needs derives from a fragmented and partial understanding of the relation between the individual patients, health care providers, and those governmental and industrial organizations that attempt to serve them. As Strauss notes:

> Chronically ill people, low in energy, with mobility problems and difficult regimen schedules and the like, are often hard put to get to certain facilities and at the institutionally scheduled times. Moreover, the sources of information that they or any other sick person—but especially they—need about available services are far from adequate.[2]

Information concerning the needs of patients is somehow cut off from those organizations and policy makers who determine the manner in which care is delivered.

Where, in research or professional studies, do we find the patient's view of his or her own illness? Little appears in the literature that describes ESRD from the patient's perspective. As a result, the patient's perspective does not often become part of economic, technical, or health policy decision making. Information is controlled and filtered by the physicians and the unit staff. Patients are generally curious about new clinical findings and policy issues but have limited access to this information.[3]

There are, however, groups who claim to represent ESRD patients. The National Kidney Foundation is concerned with the cost and quality of care in the ESRD treatment and constitutes a vocal interest group in controversies with the government, particularly those surrounding proposed legislative changes that affect the treatment program. Other organizations, representing the voice of physicians involved with renal care and transplantation, are the Renal Physicians Association and the American Society of Transplant Surgeons. The National Association for Patients on Hemodialysis and Transplantation, on the other hand, has worked in conjunction with the National Kidney Foundation to lobby strenuously for inclusion of payment for treatment services, again under the Social Security amendment.

Additional organizations have been established, but the extent to which they permeate the barriers of constructive communication and advocate change on the behalf of the patients, staff, and family alike is difficult to assess. Journals, notably *Dialysis and Transplantation*, also provide information to professionals and patients. In interviews at one treatment program I found that fewer than 35 percent of the patients subscribed to publications or enrolled in clubs or organizations representing ESRD patients.

A variety of perspectives compete with a patient-oriented understanding of ESRD. Health policy debates, legislation, clinical research, and the bioengineering industry all contribute to the social construction of ESRD. These perspectives influence the nature of health care service to ESRD patients and affect their families and health care professionals in diverse ways. For example, from the perspective of federal health policy makers, we find that ESRD holds a unique status within the government: it is the first and only disease for which treatment costs are covered for nearly all afflicted persons, regardless of age or income. Therefore, a disproportionate amount of attention is paid to the costs of this one disease.[4] Congressional efforts to reduce health care costs always seem to highlight the ESRD program. Government efforts are under way to monitor and contain costs, which by 1984 reached nearly $2 billion per year for treatment expenditures. Legislation and regulatory efforts to lessen the pace of unnecessary program growth in any federal entitlement program is reasonable. Because ESRD treatment involves diverse ethical, social, and economic issues, an effective policy for the delivery and payment of services to ESRD patients seems particularly difficult.[5] The complexity of the public perspective centers on the following issues:

1. The major treatment modalities, hemodialysis and transplantation, are the only life-saving alternatives for ESRD patients, yet

they have gained that status without exploration of the question of *adequacy of treatment* through empirical testing, i.e., randomized clinical trials. Reasonable assurance that these techniques prolonged life apparently was the sole clinical criterion of success.

2. The denial of treatment for any ESRD patient was considered unethical; therefore, the government proceeded to pass legislation mandating that all patients be treated, regardless of age, financial status, or appropriateness of techniques for the patients. The result has been a great increase in the average severity of illness of ESRD patients. (See Chapter 7.)

3. Anyone having ESRD qualifies for Medicare, and the price of treatment is not set in a "free" market. The U.S. government is the largest, if not the sole, consumer of ESRD service. As a consequence, the economic characters of such a system are poorly understood.

4. The impetus behind federal funding of a special treatment program for ESRD patients was to establish a cost-effective technology, available to all, that would also have a rehabilitative impact; that is, one that would return persons with chronic renal failure to economic productivity.[6] Despite these hopes, rehabilitation efforts have had limited effects. Private industry has no incentive to employ, rehire, or retrain those patients who might be able to return to work part time.

5. The costs (to the federal government) associated with the established ESRD treatments (in ascending order) are transplantation, home dialysis, and in-center or hospital-based dialysis, respectively. In-center dialysis, however, was chosen more often by physicians and patients because there had been a financial disincentive for home care. Also, home care is not appropriate for many patients for a variety of reasons.

6. Industrial and medical-center research is based almost entirely on ESRD treatment, rather than on prevention or early detection.

7. CAPD is a new, supposedly less costly treatment for ESRD. It is, however, in its experimental stages, and though it has met with some short-term successes, many of the long-term problems need to be addressed and technical improvements made before it is added to the list of treatment regimens for a large segment of the ESRD population. Preliminary evidence indicates that complications increase in CAPD.[7]

This complex policy milieu (which I will consider at length in Part II) suggests a great deal of uncertainty in which decisions are made, often without a careful consideration of their multiple, although difficult-to-measure, effects on the dynamics of patient experience. Dollars spent somehow become a more "real" problem than quality or appropriate care. ESRD providers deliver care with these "policy" concerns as a constant pressure on their activities and decision making.

The Health Care Providers' Perspective

Chronic illness provides a special challenge to health care providers. Strauss, delineating the difference between acute and chronic disease and between cure and care, suggests that the differences represent "something of a paradox so characteristic of contemporary health care."[8] Health care providers who consider chronic disease an important problem all too often define issues surrounding chronic disease from within an acute disease framework. The training of these professionals stresses the recovery of the patient in a framework largely influenced by a curative medical approach.

As Strauss points out, taking a strictly categorical approach to chronic illness allows us to miss too much. He argues against this approach for two reasons: First, to treat medical problems of any chronically ill patient, one must supplement the strictly medical knowledge with psychological and social knowledge about the patient and the patient's milieu. Second, because chronically ill patients share many psychological and social problems, an understanding of these can facilitate efforts to improve these patients' lives.

Chronic illness can erect many obstacles to a normal lifestyle. The key problems faced by the chronically ill in their daily lives are:
1. Preventing medical crises and managing them once they occur.
2. Controlling symptoms.
3. Carrying out of prescribed regimens and managing attendant problems.
4. Preventing or living with social isolation.
5. Adjusting to changes in the course of the disease, whether it moves downward or enters a period of remission.
6. Attempting to keep interaction with others and style of life as normal as possible.

7. Finding the necessary money—to pay for treatments or to survive despite partial or complete loss of employment.
8. Managing the *physician's work*, that is, actively creating a context of care and treatment that has meaning.[9]

Health care providers perform the four I's: informing, interceding, interpreting, and instructing. In many cases their role goes beyond the strictly medical services provided to these chronically ill patients. They *inform* patients about new medical technologies, alternative treatment; they *intercede* or represent patients in issues involving not only the members of the medical staff itself but also the patient's social and economic support systems; they *interpret* social/health policy and attitudes to the patients; and, finally, they *instruct* patients and their families in self-care techniques, and the rationale and methods of the treatment regimens. Through these actions the health care providers become a part of the patient's illness experience and profoundly affect not only the patient, but also family, friends, donors, and, ultimately, the public perspective on the medical event.

The renal unit staff is often not aware of their power or their limitations. In fact, the staff often deny their involvement in the illness experience and attempt to blame or defer responsibility to the patient or family when problems do arise. A number of studies have observed this type of staff denial.[10] But I am suggesting that there is an additional "meta-denial" by those who research the psychosocial factors of ESRD that compounds this problem and that, in fact, legitimates staff denial. Nemiah defines denial as a "mechanism of defense in which the facts or logical implications of external reality are refused recognition in favor of internally derived, wish-fulfilling fantasies."[11] Much of the current research on ESRD patients exhibits just such denial of, or at least "selective inattention" to, the full range of complex issues that patients must face and to the staff-patient conflict that often results. This is not to say that such research does not contribute to our understanding of the illness experience in ESRD. It is, rather, that such lines of inquiry are often limited by their reliance on psychoanalytic classifications of symptoms and by their focus on a narrow range of social aspects of chronic renal failure, that is, adaptation to transplantation. This limited perspective on the social aspects of ESRD presents an unbalanced account of the problem. The importance of the social dynamics *among* the patient, the staff, and the physician is ignored or denied, and the conflicts are often said to have their source in the patient's personality (the "non-compliance" label) or a "deficient" family's lack of support.

Conflicts between the staff and patients are inherent in ESRD treatment. These can be described as a network of conflicting and shifting expectations. Sometimes independence is expected of patients and is encouraged. At the same time, too much independence is considered a problem (noncompliance). Resentment of a patient, particularly an independent one, is exacerbated by the treatment staff's lingering sense of powerlessness in treating a complex and terminal illness.

In perhaps the most widely read description of these issues, Fox and Swazey give the impression that nephrologists and transplant surgeons do not have a problematic role in ESRD treatment. In their account, the dynamics of the clinic are simple; they reduce patients to helpless beneficiaries and elevate physicians to courageous risk-takers. Fox and Swazey present patients as uncomfortable in their physical illness and psychological guilt; they often "cannot do enough to appreciate what the physician has done for them."[12] Moreover, the patient who does not comply in the "sick role" is basically undeserving of the "Gift." Of course, Fox and Swazey compliment patients, particularly the transplant patients, by noting that the transplant physicians and research teams consider them to be "esteemed and heroic companions in a perilous but promising group endeavor that makes 'front line' kindred of all participants."[13] They do not recognize that the transplant patient plays a special role in the ideology of ESRD treatment. A successful transplant patient is "cured" and therefore represents the clearest legitimation of ESRD technology. In fact, successful transplantation for a large segment of the ESRD population has been the major unfulfilled promise of this technology.[14] Further, the "kinship network" they describe is both temporary and ideological—the failed transplant patient quickly returns to the rank and file when the transplant fails.

When one thinks of the integral role the patient's attitude has in overall recovery and rehabilitation, one must ask, why shouldn't all patients be treated as if they were working members of the treatment team? Why is this not an expectation of quality ESRD care? In the traditional Parsonian model used by Fox and Swazey, patients are assigned to "sick roles." Their behavior is judged by the extent to which they conform to the established norms of this role. The patient has a circumscribed place in the ceremonial order of the renal clinic, a place that is epiphenomenal to the scientific ritual of treatment.

This framework also influences other "professional" views of the problem of ESRD. The literature is replete with articles that attempt to classify the norms of compliance or noncompliance of ESRD patients. Some researchers develop their norms within a psychoanalytic framework.[15] Others attempt to typologize behavior in medical terms, as Calland notes.[16] Still others focus on narrow aspects of the chronic renal disease, such as studies on transplantation.[17]

In these writings, the framework presents nephrologists, dialysis teams, and transplant surgeons as ideal types. For example, in carrying out what Fox and Swazey call gatekeeping functions, the physicians must screen who will and who will not be adequate donors— who will be able to take part in the exchange of the gift. The final gatekeeper is the physician. As they see it:

> The physician is acting on the behalf of the transplant team, the patient, and possibly donors and their relatives, as well as for himself; he makes the ultimate judgement. The physician's role here is as sociological and moral as it is medical. He acts as mediator and interpreter in the complex social system called into play by the transplantation situation. In this capacity, he weaves his way back and forth among the patient, candidate donors, their families, and the wide range of specialists who constitute the transplantation team. His role here is like that of the superior of a religious order who, in the name of high ethical and spiritual values, controls what gifts can be offered and received by the members of the community he represents. The physician is not free to abrogate his responsibility, nor may he exercise it arbitrarily or coercively. He must base his decision on biomedical, psychological, and sociological criteria that are acceptable within his profession.[18]

What criteria are applied and what constitutes an acceptable decision within the professional peer group? Is this such a simple decision framework for a nephrologist? Certainly there are contradictory forces within these criteria, as the nephrologist is often negotiating multiple professional roles: care provider, researcher, and teacher, among others.

In contrast, Czackes and Kaplan-DeNour present an alternative to godlike images of nephrologists that Fox and Swazey present.[19] From a psychoanalytic perspective, they recognize that the quality of the interaction between physicians and patient and poor management of these tensions adversely affect patients. However, the problem of the socially deficient patient is transferred to the patient's personality structure itself. The implication of this, of course, is that the patient is again blamed for the problem, but this time for not having the ego defenses to prevent serious psychopathological consequences. Conversely, the patient must have come into the clinical context with existing psychological problems that exacerbate the difficulties experienced in dialysis.

More socially oriented researchers like Halper or O'Brien have recognized that a staff's work in a dialysis unit is a rewarding experience when things go well but a much more difficult one when things go wrong.[20] The staff, consisting of a few technicians and nurses, a dietician, a supervising physician (a nephrologist or a transplant surgeon), a social worker, and some additional personnel, works with a small number of patients and has intensive contact with them for long periods. Surprisingly, the physician has the least contact with the patients; the nurses and technicians, the most. The technicians and nurses, then, learn most about the patients' lives and must deal with their families; they maintain long-term relationships, become more involved with the patient's fears and hopes, and watch the patient develop complications and die.

In the dialysis unit, the death of a patient takes on a special significance. It is, on the one hand, acknowledged as an important loss to the staff, but there is a conflict when it is clearly a case in which the patient wanted to die, despite the staff's contrary desire.[21] The option of "dying with dignity" is undoubtedly a major legal, ethical, and psychological issue in the dialysis unit.

Simmons et al. also represent a more sociological framework (as opposed to the psychoanalytic one), focusing on the physician's perception of the transplant patient.[22] In this study, the majority of patients and families for whom the transplant was successful coped well with stress and exhibited some long-term gains from having successfully survived their enormous crisis. Physicians' feelings and perceptions about those patients who are *not* to experience transplants were different. The study, exhaustive as it is in presenting psychosocial dynamics derived from surveys or interviews, reports only the small number of "successful" transplants. The "social factors," then, primarily reflect the physician's relationship or view of what makes a successful transplant patient. These factors for social success are:

1. That class background may affect a patient's chances to be referred for transplantation.
2. That social factors governing the dissemination of accurate information concerning medical innovations, and the interrelationships between centralized medical institutions and referring physicians, play a large role in whether a patient will get a transplant.
3. That the role of the local/referring physician is crucial in the case of transplantation, since this physician is generally the one who first approaches the family with the suggestion of donation.
4. That the referring/local community physician's professional network, knowledge about transplants, and awareness of the types of patients that are suited for transplant all play a critical role in whether or not the patient will be referred.[23]

The social question seems bounded by a clinical definition of a successful transplant and the generalized, optimistic attitude that transplant surgeons have toward their patients. The staff's perception of patients is often the cause of the patients' problems, and not merely the result of them.

These studies demonstrate how the conventional wisdom of the clinical perspective becomes incorporated into social and psychological research frameworks. Although these studies present themselves as external or evaluative analyses, they in fact adopt the clinical perception of the "needs" of ESRD patients. The social or behavioral scientists seem to share the gaze of the clinicians. They are "doctors" in spite of themselves.

The Response of the Family to the ESRD Patient

Studies of the family or social supports of ESRD patients also have a characteristic orientation. Relatives, spouses, or donors are rarely the authors; instead, they are the subjects of analyses written by psychiatrists or social science researchers. And little psychosocial research has focused on the patient's social network.[24] As Simmons discussed, most of what is written considers the spouse of the patient in home care, especially since he or she is usually the primary caretaker. Hence, the marital and sexual relations and family role issues become the focus of analysis. The issues less often discussed are those relating to the broader social networks of patients. How does the downward illness trajectory of ESRD and the possibility of death influence a range of experiences in social life beyond the context of the traditional family? Such questions are not the major concerns of the family support studies.

The hidden costs to the family, that is, the lack of income due to the patient's unemployment or day-care costs, are often sources of resentment and anger in the patient's family, particularly in the spouse of the ESRD patient, and pose a set of difficult problems. The sick role is often extended to include the primary caretaker when, for example, the spouse "fails" to cooperate or "gives in" to the pressures of the treatment protocols. Spouses are portrayed in research studies as noncompliant or selfish and may even be labeled as having a personality disorder.

Some examples of studies looking at the marital relations of "dialysis couples" include a study by Finkelstein, which assessed and rated marital problems.[25] This study found close agreement between patient and spouse in their ratings of marital problems. Finkelstein also compared the *researcher's* evaluation of the couples' marital relations and, interestingly enough, found that they perceived more discord than the couples did. Finkelstein suggested that the patients' depression may be a significant contributing factor to the couples' sexual problems.

Santopietro found that dialysis couples may be stigmatized by friends and relatives because of the patients' unusual treatment regimen; therefore, they must often rely on the treatment team for support and encouragement.[26] This study emphasized that spouses have "unconscious hostility," perhaps even "homicidal impulses," toward the dialysis patient and that the wives of these patients frequently experienced a loss of self-esteem and sense of identity as a woman, wife, and mother that began with their husbands' illness. No social or contextual analysis of these findings is presented.

Regardless of the treatment chosen (home or in-center dialysis treatment), the immediate family, relatives, and friends of a patient will inevitably be affected. Although home dialysis is less expensive in terms of direct costs to the federal government, its social costs to the patient and family can be high. When one family member treats another with a life-saving technology that has even a small potential for failure, the stress can be significant. Even in those studies that report favorable family adaptation, it is still noted that those with a higher quality of interaction to begin with generally fare better in maintaining a more healthful, emotionally stable environment for the patient.[27] That is, if the social support is strong before the onset of ESRD, the patient's outcome will be better. Social support may, in fact, be the most important prognostic variable, all other things being equal.

It is difficult to assess the long-term effects on the families, friends, and relatives of ESRD patients from the research on stress in ESRD. Most of the psychosocial research does not consider the dynamic nature of such a mutually interactive social system. The social scientists seem to be paradigmatically aligned with their clinical counterparts, restricted by the simple individuality of the medical model.

Patient Experience—Psychiatric Labeling versus Grounded Discovery

How can we begin to understand the patient's experience without the encumbrances of the medical or psychosocial model? The majority of what is reported about patients' perceptions of ESRD is drawn from psychiatric reports, staff unit surveys, patient surveys, and case studies that depend on those models for their framework. What is presented, therefore, is an interpretation of what the patient feels or thinks, mediated by the researchers conducting the study. The studies inadvertently tell more about themselves than about their subjects. We therefore learn more about the problems of this particular way of framing patient experience than we add to our understanding of actual patient experience.

One approach to understanding the patients' own experience and perception of chronic renal failure might center on those issues related to his or her quality of life, as the patient defines it. However, much of the current research on quality focuses on psychiatric symptomatology or measurable adverse clinical conditions. In evaluating the psychological status of an ESRD patient, the physician, psychologist, social worker, or nurse confronts symptoms that may appear on the one hand to be functional in origin but, on the other hand, may result from the patient's organic disorder or be a combination of both. This fact causes great uncertainty for the professional providing mental health services to the ESRD patient. For example, the patient may complain of drowsiness, apathy, and inability to concentrate, but it is difficult for the psychiatrist (looking for a specific cause) to determine if it is due to depression, to organic brain syndrome (as a result of the patient's uremia), or to both. Although etiology is a moot point for the patient who experiences these symptoms, it is not for the attending psychiatrist, who must determine what treatment to employ. The presenting psychological symptoms of any ESRD patient are usually the consequences of interacting physiological, social, and psychological stresses. Despite the widely varied psychological effects these stresses can cause, ESRD patients' responses are labeled according to traditional psychiatric nosology.

The most frequently reported behavioral symptom is depression. Patients complain of extreme anxiety and fear of death, apathy, extreme dependency needs, denial, sleep disorders, inability to concentrate, fatigue, and suicidal tendencies.[28] Suicide is thought to be about 400 percent higher in ESRD patients than in the general population.[29] Organic brain syndrome, generally a complication of uremia, is also commonly cited in the literature. Some of its specific symptoms are drowsiness, apathy, attentional problems, and slurred and slowed speech. These symptoms persist as long as the uremia does, and hence are not a sign of permanent deterioration.[30] Other symptoms reported in ESRD patients include anger and hostility, aggression, delusions, hallucinations, and paranoid and psychotic behaviors.

These correspond to the major categories of psychiatric labeling; they are recognizable and form coherent categories for the psychiatrist. But the social nexus of ESRD patients that influences such symptomatology and the patients' own definitions of the illness experience form a separate reality.

What life stresses of the ESRD patient are discussed in the "observer" studies? Wright et al. divided the psychological stresses of hemodialysis into three groups: (1) actual or threatened losses: of body functions, of jobs, of money; (2) injury or the threat of injury, i.e., from surgical procedures; and (3) the frustration of instinctual drives: extreme dietary restrictions, sexual dysfunction.[31]

These stresses manifest themselves in many ways. Anger and aggression are perhaps the most difficult ones for patients to express and for staff to deal with. Halper addresses this issue of anger: it is hard for the patient to express anger toward a "miraculous process" that gives him "life" three times a week or toward the conscientious staff that takes care of him but may also cause him pain. The patient feels guilt and fears retaliation if he directly expresses his anger.[32] Frequently, this anger is internalized and expressed toward the self through a suicide attempt. Abrams has found that many patients express anger through suicidal attempts. For Abrams, noncompliance is roughly equivalent to suicide; there is no social context for noncompliance; a patient either follows directions or does not.[33] Halper takes a different position, that it is "natural" for the ESRD patient to contemplate suicide. He encourages expression of those feelings. He emphasizes, however, that the patient indeed has something to live for and should be encouraged to recognize this.[34]

Although most of the information about the patient's perspective is based on reports of symptoms by psychiatrically oriented researchers, there are a few exceptions. Charles Calland, a physician and ESRD patient who had experienced numerous transplantations and dialyses, has written from his unique perspective of the illness.[35] His sensitive account emphasized the inconsistencies between what is conventionally understood to be the day-to-day reality of chronic renal failure in research studies and the experience of ESRD patients. In contrast to what is generally discussed in the literature, Calland views the patient's fear or "depression" as being far more grounded in the social context of ESRD treatment than is usually recognized. Patients fear the accidental unplugging of the machine, the financial burden that their families must encounter, and stigmatization by their friends as a result of their "marginal existence."[36] Rather than viewing the patient as a victim who deserves blame for being unable to cope with stresses, Calland appreciates the social disruption caused by serious chronic diseases and, importantly, the isolation that the patient confronts both in the clinical setting and in the broader social context. He asks the questions that few providers ever consider: is ESRD treatment the best answer for all patients with kidney failure? He calls attention to how frequently the patient is made to feel marginal in the clinical setting. Physicians control critical information and are reluctant to communicate this with patients, particularly those who are not showing progress. This insider's view, by a person who knows both "cultures" of the clinical relationship, the professional's and patient's, presents the problems of the root metaphor of the "psychosocial" approach to ESRD.

Transplantation presents a special case in any analysis of the patient's experience in ESRD. A transplantable kidney that becomes available to the patient is viewed as "the gift of life," the ultimate technical promise, a chance to return to the "nondiseased" state. The initial psychological adjustment to the transplant, assuming it is successful, is much easier than the initial adjustment to long-term renal dialysis. Special problems do exist initially. For example, with cadaver donors, the patient may experience some distortions of body image, or in the case of a relative-donor, the relationship between the patient and donor before the surgery will usually dictate adjustment postoperatively.[37] However, the ease of adjustment rests on the certainty of rejection, but at an unknown time. When the transplant fails, readjustment to dialysis is often extremely difficult.

Divergent Goals and Expectations—From Clinical Uncertainty to Federal Policy

Thus far we have explored some of the prevailing incongruous expectations that characterize various research perspectives in ESRD. Although home dialysis appears more economical for the patient than in-center care, the psychological costs paid by both the patient and the family are often greater, even though the patient may exercise more autonomy. Although transplantation is the least expensive (for the federal government and patient) and represents a "cure," it also has significant medical risks and a high probability of failure. Moreover, donors (cadaver or living) are not easily found.

The federal government pays for most of the treatment costs for most patients under the assumption that these individuals will be successfully rehabilitated and return to economic productivity in the community. This has overwhelmingly not proven to be the reality for most ESRD patients.[38] Reimbursement policies also do not consider many hidden costs of illness: child care, limited potential to acquire gainful employment, the difficulty of performing a range of social activities, and the psychological traumas of terminal illness. The government provides no incentives for private industry to rehire, retrain, or maintain on a part-time basis those patients who are healthy enough to work. Firms who produce medical technology, influenced by the drive toward greater profitability in the dialysis market, also carry problematic assumptions that shape the context of patient care. These two powerful forces, industry and government, ensure that changes in the prevailing notions of "effective" service delivery will not come easily. This is particularly the case as the federal government maintains its status as the sole payer for services. The old adage "He who pays the piper calls the tune" applies here. The federal government sings one tune: cost control. Notions like quality of care, the experience of illness, and a social perspective on ESRD treatment policy are too complex for the federal payer.

This backing away from the social complexity of ESRD by the federal government influences the conflicts that arise in the dialysis unit between patients and physicians and between the unit's staff, the patient, and the family. It is here that the issues of dependency-independence, quality versus quantity of life, denial on the part of both patients and staff, miscommunication and noncommunication, and the technology of hope come into focus. As a result of their training, physicians and clinical staff members are inclined to view the ideal patient as one who concedes to their demands and requirements, complies with the treatment regimen, trusts in their professional competence, can cope with the stress in his illness, all without involving the provider unduly in the patient's personal affairs outside the clinic. The patient should also be optimistic and motivated toward rehabilitation. Although these are perhaps laudable goals, such expectations may, for many chronic renal disease patients, be unrealistic or explicitly inappropriate. Psychiatrists' belief that it is "natural" for ESRD patients to feel suicidal presents a strong indication that the context of care for ESRD patients might itself be pathological, particularly in a social sense.

Imagine the patient who is assertive, independent, impervious to pain and discomfort, strong-willed in keeping to a diet, thoughtful and appreciative of every newly applied shunt, and relieved and content about no longer being able to attain career goals or to maintain personal and family relationships. This, given the current context of ESRD, would be quite "deviant." The point is, the criteria for what is normal and what is deviant must be redefined and negotiated in the social context of actual treatment by the staff and the patient. Clearly constructed goals and expectations must be set, but with an awareness of the needs of a specific person and not according to an ideal clinical model of the patient.

CHAPTER FOUR

"Success" and "Failure"
Portraits of Health in Illness

To move from a discussion of the interactive dynamics in ESRD treatment to a more detailed look at patients' experience of illness, we must take the problems we have already discussed and extend the viewing frame to include the broader social context. What is it like to live with this life-altering disease? Who is the person behind the patient role, and what are the social contexts and personal histories into which the disease has come? What are the hopes, fears, aspirations, and concerns of the people who live with a more acute awareness of mortality and physical limitations than the rest of us?

The body of writings concerned with the experience of illness is growing at such a rate that it would have been possible to devote this book to this one subject.[1] From the many hours of interviews with patients and their families who shared their experience, some common themes emerge.

The social texture of survival is one of the most important themes. This differs from the clinical and psychosocial models of survival that have been discussed in preceding chapters. In fact, the term *survival* does not capture fully the dimension I am describing. What emerges through in the diverse life stories contained in the interviews has almost transcendental properties, will and spirit. You will find no metabolic correlates to measure will and no regression model to assess spirit, but it is these elusive, nonquantifiable characteristics that provide the courage to survive. At the core of the illness experi-

86

ence is the urge to make life meaningful, and the strategies and structure of a meaningful life are as varied as the persons who pursue the struggle.

I want to examine the process by which meaning in the context of life altered by ESRD is generated. Two portraits are presented, both largely sketched by the individuals themselves. One is of Bill Charles, who was considered a successful patient by his care providers. The other, Karen Eliot, was labeled unsuccessful by her physicians and nurses. Both of them struggled to live their lives with meaning and dignity, given their illness and social conditions.

A "Successful" Patient

Bill Charles was the person the staff described most often as the best example of a successful patient. Their wishful attitude was expressed in the question, "Why can't we have more patients like Bill?" Physicians and nurses alike were deeply impressed by this man's ability to manage his life and his disease, although they were not quite sure how he was able to do it. During my discussions with Bill, I tried to understand the social context of his illness experience and his notion of success in ESRD treatment. Our discussions also included his wife, and some of the comments that follow represent her perspective and role in making a life-threatening situation meaningful.

Bill was forty years old and working as a construction worker and truck driver when his kidneys failed. Married and the father of seven children, he had known for five years that his kidneys were failing, so it did not come as a complete surprise when he finally required dialysis. He had been treated for five years when we began our discussions.

From the start he tackled the mechanics of therapy assertively with a desire to master the technique required to control his machine-assisted life.

I really didn't have problems starting off with it. I mean I wasn't too appreciative of going on that, but I knew that it was something that I had to face. I didn't do too bad—the first couple of days I put my own needles in. And the doctor was quite pleased with it because usually it took longer for a patient to do the needles. I just said I've got to do it—I might as well do it. I think it's mainly your own attitude—that you're willing to accept—well, like for example, you can be doing anything, whether it's a kidney machine or not—your life is that if you have a failure—well you don't just stop, you just turn around and pick yourself up and find another way to go around the mountain, under the mountain, over the mountain or whichever way you want to do. That's basically in your own mind.

Cathy, Bill's wife, added:

Well, it's not anything anybody would choose, of course. But it's a matter of accepting what comes. You just have to live with it and you make it part of your routine and that's all. I must say the first day that I went in for training I came home in a state of shock. Because being an R.N. I really thought that I ought to know the machine. But, at the time that I was still working, they didn't even have machines. So after that, it came a little easier. We didn't have any difficulties learning the mechanics of it and with a medical background, I think it makes it a little easier. Although there are many people who do very well without any medical background.

The Charleses talked extensively about their family's experience of ESRD. Their seven children, ranging in age from four to sixteen, were an important part of the family's adaptation to the demands of Bill's illness. They had chosen home dialysis, and two of their older boys assisted their father on the dialysis machine from the very beginning. Bill and Cathy made an effort to integrate the process of dialysis into their interaction with the children. The machine was not thought of as "other" or something separate from "family space." The tasks related to Bill's dialysis therapy became a focus for family activity. As Cathy said:

From the very beginning we've allowed them . . . taught them how to do blood pressure. We've taught them how to monitor all the gauges. A couple of them even give him his weekly injections. So they've always been part of it and they just take it right in their stride as just part of their life. Their friends—when they come up—get a little upset sometimes.

Although they both believed that this sharing of responsibility for dialysis was generally a positive thing for their family, the arrangement was not without problems.

They really like to show off to their friends. But they've taken it well. I think the younger ones may have been a little fearful because of a number of things that have happened. Of course, the older ones are more aware of the possibilities—of things that might happen. He had innumerable viruses, whatever came along, he caught. And he went from over 200 pounds to 140 and couldn't walk because of the pain and for a couple of weeks couldn't even sleep upstairs—had to sleep on the chair downstairs. . . . So the kids seeing him in this condition were— he'd be home for a week-end and he'd be in for two or three months—maybe he'd be home for a few more days and he'd be in again. It was hard on them.

One time particularly I remember when Michael came home— we had had a power failure. Something went wrong. So I just called the Fire Department. I wasn't about to leave Bill and go look. So I called them. Well, they sent the fire engine. They sent the emergency truck. They sent two ambulances. They had police cars. And Michael came home from school and saw all this paraphernalia and it really hit him. He was scared to death. And we've had a couple of times when we've had to rush Bill in. I think the hemorrhages that he used to have upset them more because it was graphic. Something that's bothering you that doesn't show too much maybe isn't as frightening as blood all over the place.

Still, with all of the possible adverse events related to treatment, Bill never considered switching his dialysis treatment to hospital-based sessions. He believed that the experience brought him closer to his children.

I wanted to be with my family. This has really made it nice—doing it in the home because, you know, the kids come home from school and I'm on the machine—they come up here and my little guy— four years old—he sits right there and has his lunch. And I've gotten to know this one here, the little girl, and the three youngest better than I know my older ones because I'm with them all the time. With the others I wasn't, because they were younger and I was always out working. Now these here, my gosh, I mean like I couldn't be without them because they're so close to me.

Bill had tried kidney transplantation during the first year his kidneys failed. The transplant lasted less than a year, a period during which he experienced most of the problems and complications he has yet encountered as an ESRD patient. He did not see another transplantation as a possibility and was content with dialysis.

Since then I have sort of just backed away from a kidney transplant because just from reading and learning about transplants—second transplants are not always as good as the first one. So I said, "No I am perfectly happy on my machine and if someday I decide—I'm still young enough to go for another one." But I think basically that I have adapted my whole life around this machine. So I fit my whole life schedule to doing the machine and I've got accustomed to knowing exactly what I have to do and what I don't have to do and what my limitations are. So I am pretty well satisfied here cause it's best—it does a good job. I'm in pretty good shape compared to a lot of fellows that are on dialysis. A lot of people don't believe I'm on a kidney machine because—when they see me running around they say, "Well there's nothing wrong with you. You're perfectly healthy." But I take care of myself. I try to eat the right stuff and I try to dialyze the way I should. I try to get exercise. That's important. And it's also important—the thing is that what you put in up here—your mental attitude. And once you get a good mental attitude about it, I think you can accomplish almost anything, really, and it's just the way you happen to look at it. So basically that's the way we've handled it.

What seems at the center of Bill's strategy for success is gaining control over his treatment. He did this actively by managing both his own dialysis and the activities of health professionals responsible for his case. He was someone to be reckoned with where his treatment was involved and did not accept medical authority at face value. Bill recounted several examples of this "take charge" attitude.

Yeah, cause, you see, the thing is, I have had cases where they got a new doctor in there and I was really doing well. And the doctor came in and said, "Oh well, we've got a new medication now on the market and you gotta take it and get on this three times a day." And I went, "No way, man. I don't care what kind of a doctor you are. You get me authorization on new medicine, okay, I'll take it, I'll try it." So he called the pharmacy to tell them to order it. The pharmacy said, "We never heard of it." I went right to Dr. Haskins and I said, "Wait a minute, I don't mind taking things and trying things but I don't try something that isn't even in the hospital pharmacy. Now come on, you'd better get rid of this character." And they never let that doctor see me again because he was giving medication that really—I don't think they knew about—I never did see him around there after that either.

I've gotten several new different doctors and right away they read your chart and say, "Oh, you're on this medication and this medication. Well, maybe if you took this you might. . . ." There's no way—I'm not taking it. I feel fine. I think I should be the one to judge. As long as I feel well, why should I change the medication? Otherwise, if you took one look at me and took one look at some other patients over there, then maybe that other patient is not—is doing well on the medication that they're taking. And I'm not taking a lot of other medications. I'm only taking folic acid and a vitamin and an iron pill.

In the realm of finances and family economics, Bill and his family came up against pressures that perhaps were more difficult to control than the clinical aspects of ESRD treatment. Like the vast majority of ESRD patients, Bill—and his family—found money to be a problem. Even with Bill's strong desire to do things for himself, the conventional world of finance and employment proved too difficult to adjust to his special needs.

I'll give you an example how things work—a lot of people don't understand this—here I have a house that has not that much of a mortgage on it, but because I'm not working—I'm not actually employed in a J-O-B job—I could not even get five dollars from the bank because I am not employed. Now that's ridiculous. We wanted to remortgage our home to help straighten out our bills and things like this. They said, "Oh no, sorry, you're not employed." I went out even to get a job—I can go to work five or six hours a day—and you know what they told me?—"Sorry, we can't hire you, you're a risk." Now the employer was willing to hire me, but the insurance company said, "Sorry, we can't cover that man—he's a risk." Like they'll say to you, "Why don't you go back to work?" How can I go back to work? I go try to work and the guy wants to hire me but the insurance company says, "No way." See, that's when things have to really get dug into and start learning that people do need help and I think it's an injustice for an insurance company to collect insurance and money and everything like this and not be on the helping end, only on the taking end. They're really a gross injustice to society that way.

That is really a burden. I mean really because you see—I can give you an example in my case. I have seven children. . . . I sent my kids over here to [a Catholic] school. Now I took care of my kids' education before I had the kidney problem. But now see I owe the school over here $2,000 for my kids' education. So they just sent me a letter not too long ago saying, "Sorry, but you can't send your kids to this school no more 'cause you didn't pay your bill." So now what do I do? In other words, I can't send my kids where I would like to send them which is an injustice. They go to a parochial school over here. That's my religion, my belief. Why shouldn't I be able to educate my children the way I want to? And I think that it's a very unjust thing, and I think that's one of the biggest problems with people who are on dialysis. First of all, they are afraid to go out and make any extra money because, for the simple reason, the Social Security will cut them off and they can't afford to lose what they've already got. So it's like saying, "Okay, you be a good boy and you just do what you're supposed to do and just manage." And that's a tough thing to do.

For many patients in his situation (an eighth-grade education, a job history of heavy, manual work, and large family-related expenses), the inability to find work and the dehumanizing maze of disability entitlement programs are too much. It is understandable that many ESRD patients cannot bear the pressure, become depressed, and slowly lose the will and spirit to struggle against the burden of illness. Certainly, the national data on "rehabilitation" attests to the difficulty of integrating meaningful and gainful work into the life experience of ESRD.

Bill, however, was the exceptional patient. When confronted with the problem of money, he tried a different strategy.

I was going back to finish up my high school education because I didn't finish my education. It sort of bothered me that I wasn't equipped with an education that I could go do a job that I might do. So I pondered over that a while and then I just said, "Oh, forget it, I've got more brains in my head than most people got whether they got an education or not, and I can do anything I want to do." It's all what I make up my mind to do. And since then I've just got into this business and I've been doing fantastic.

Well, our business is very lucrative and we are really developing a good income. And what we're doing now is—see I can't travel. So, but with my business being lucrative like this, I am in the process now of buying a motor coach—a big motor coach. Then I'm going to install a kidney machine in the coach, and then I can travel and dialyze. I can go across the country. See my business is not just here. My business is worldwide. So I can go anywhere I want in the world and work. I deal with people. I don't deal with products as much. I train people that are not satisfied with their present day income how to establish a second income or a permanent business.

Cathy was also involved in this "business," which they discussed in stages, not wanting to tell me too much about it too soon. Bill addressed a few questions to me.

Hey look, would you be interested in having a business of your own—and making all the money that you could ever need, and not have to worry about it?

Because I've got a business where I've got the funds that I can travel. And that's my whole business now—is how can I help somebody else get what I've already got. And I want to tell you something—I guarantee anybody that if I could sit—anybody in the education—in your field or within—the doctors or anything—could sit down for an hour and listen to what I have to say, I would change a few people's minds. First of all, I'll give you an example. You're in what you're in because you love what you're doing. But you still need to make money to support yourself. Everybody—I don't care what you do—needs money. And the thing is—you better get your head on straight if you say you don't need it. Well then you better sit down and listen to what I have to tell you because I can make you $30,000 a year if you listen to what I tell you in 90 days. I mean I know that for a fact.

Very quickly the interviewer/subject roles had shifted, and this energetic, dynamic fellow was clearly in control of this interview, too.

One thing is that in what I have you're ignorant. You are an ignorant person really. I don't mean that as a put-down or anything. But you are an ignorant person because, you see, once I show you what I have you are no longer ignorant. The only people who don't join me and do what I have to do are ignorant people. So anything anybody has to offer, if I show it to you, then you are no longer ignorant. And then once I release it to you and I show you what it is—it's up to you—you make your choice because I don't need anybody. I don't really need anybody to become successful. I'm already successful.

After this windup, then came the pitch:

This thing that I have—that I'm connected with is the largest and fastest growing thing in the country today. This—what I'm with—started out 18 years ago. They are doing such a business. They're doing a million dollars a day and growing and totally solvent. They don't owe a dime and all's I got to do is to mention to some government official—and they can look it up—they got a triple Dun & Bradstreet A rating—4 A—and they are the leading company in the U.S. today. Dupont used to be leading. Now this company is the top thing and the only way you will find out what it is is by through me. And it is so fantastic. I'm so positive about this—that it would make you look like some magic person. "Where did you find this idea?" You want to make a name for yourself. That will make a name for you.

For the next hour Bill tried (unsuccessfully) to sell me an Amway distributorship. With a confidence bordering on hucksterism, Bill had found a way to capitalize on his vast resources of optimism and hope. He involved himself in a decentralized corporation whose success is premised on those very principles. The disability of ESRD did not diminish his efforts in this enterprise. Out of the tragedy of a catastrophic disease, Bill and Cathy used home dialysis to bring their family closer together. A family-oriented business seems to have enhanced these relations further. Bill summarized his "success" this way:

A lot of patients have decided to live a mediocre life and they don't have to. I have proven that. Because I could have lived a mediocre life—I could have laid back and said, "Okay, everybody, take care of me." But I had seven little ones here that said, "Hey, that's not fair. You brought us into the world, now keep moving." I can't do the things that I used to do—a lot of things that I would love to do, like go on and play basketball maybe—because I don't have the energy that way. But my kids still love me for what I am and what I can be to them.

I have in my existence touched a lot of people—because I'll go to a function, and when they find out that I'm on dialysis they want to know all about it. And they just say, "It's amazing. You look like you do and you're so positive and you're doing things. Why is it that we can't do it because we're perfectly healthy?" It's your mental attitude. You have to believe yourself and believe in what you're doing. It's just like when you're doing your work, you have to believe it or forget it—you might as well quit it. And that's what people have to understand that you do not get success unless you believe and motivate yourself. I don't look at this thing here as a problem. I just look at it that it was a blessing in disguise for me because I have learned to accept what I had to accept. And the only difficult thing that I had found was the fact of not having the income to support the family at that point. That's why I had to go out and make the income so that I could be self-supporting. That's basically it in a nutshell.

A "Problem" Patient

Karen Eliot was a twenty-nine-year-old black woman with a small, almost frail constitution. Her hair had begun to gray, making her appear even older. Her manner was generally subdued. She employed short, direct phrases in a straightforward manner. During many of our discussions, she was in pain and expressed her discomfort openly. Tears and extensive crying out replaced her usual parsimonious conversation. Fragile and worn, she would toss in her bed, turning away from me for a moment. When the pain subsided (if it did subside), she would turn back, somewhat exhausted and with apologies, to resume our conversation.

Until she turned twenty-three, Karen had had a normal history of personal illness. Sickness had been an important part of her family experience, as her sister has suffered from sickle-cell disease since her early teens and her father was a severe diabetic. Five years before our interviews, Karen developed a severe and rapidly progressing form of diabetes, which was controlled with some difficulty. One year later she became pregnant; against the advice of her physician, she decided to have the child.

Two years after the birth of her son, she developed the first symptoms of renal disease. Initial attempts to manage fluid buildups and uremia with diuretics met with no success, and her kidney function diminished rapidly. Karen "woke up one day," she said, in an intensive care area being given peritoneal dialysis—an experience that had a tremendous social and psychological impact on her life. In her words:

> Everyone around me was really in a bad way—moaning and dying. I felt really uncomfortable. . . . They had a tube in my stomach and it was filled up with water and I couldn't sleep or eat. . . . Then they transferred me out to a private room and they brought the machine in there. I don't know why they put people in those private rooms. God—I hate them. . . . I don't know what it is but I really hate those private rooms.

She recounted her fears, concerns, and the changes she felt— changes in her attitude about her body, now machine-dependent; concern for her loss of appetite—she talked of how she used to be a big eater; fears about the complexity of this experience—so much could go wrong, infections, pumps, etc. After four months of this she wanted to go home.

> I was really afraid because I didn't like that peritoneal dialysis and they told me that was what I was going to have. . . . The thought of having that tube stuck out of my stomach all the time. You know, you have to be real careful with it, cleaning it and capping it up. . . . They told me they were afraid to send me home because I might get the tube infected . . . but they ran some tests and found out that I'd already got an infection [peritonitis] in the hospital. I said, hell, if I got that here, how could I be safe at home!

This ambivalence between her fear and anger concerning the faults of the hospital setting and her dependence on its technology and "safe" environment is a theme that arose often in Karen's version of her illness experience.

After this extended episode she was switched to a different treatment, hemodialysis, and had the first of a number of intravenous fistulas (to provide access for the dialysis needles) surgically constructed. Many of her fistulas failed because of problems with her venous system related to her underlying diabetic condition. She had had a generally difficult course on hemodialysis because of complications due to her diabetic condition—blood clots, hemorrhages, and extreme joint stiffness. She also developed an intolerance for the blood-clotting drug used to stop bleeding after dialysis. Because of this, she had to wait almost two hours after dialysis for her access spot to stop bleeding. Other problems such as glucose management, severe anemia requiring frequent blood transfusions, extreme puritis (itching), and transient infections have been a part of her general experience.

Some members of the treatment staff took me aside early in the course of my interviews to tell me about Karen's "psychiatric" problems. They spoke of her anger, resentment, and extreme dependence. Karen was considered quite a "patient management" problem. She was held to be a "problem" by other patients as well. A patient who often dialyzed at the same time described Karen this way: "I don't know why *anyone* would act that way." At one point Karen was referred to a psychiatrist, whom she saw a number of times. In her words:

You know, they have lots of different kinds of doctors here—too many. I can't keep them straight . . . and forget some of their names. Sometimes the psychiatrist comes around and talks to me. He asks me, "Do you hate the machine?" I thought that was a *stupid* question—I said "No, I don't hate the *machine*, the *machine* keeps me alive and I'd be dead without it. I just hate being in this hospital, . . . just don't like to have to spend all this time here."

Because of Karen's multiple medical problems she required a great deal of nursing—a situation that wore on her and on the staff. There was tension in the interactions between Karen and the nurses in the unit. As a result of all this, she was generally lethargic. When at home, she talked of being quite tired, but she had also developed a chronic difficulty in sleeping that only exacerbated her condition. Home was not a place where she could find respite from medical problems, as her diabetic condition often caused her to experience cramps, dizziness and, on occasion, blackouts.

Karen's family was an important part of her illness experience. She lived with her mother and father, an older sister and younger brother. Her sister had sickle-cell disease and had to be hospitalized four or five times a year for up to three weeks at a time. Karen took care of her sister's five-year-old son when she was in the hospital for transfusions.

Her sister's longstanding illness dominated the family. They had always had to support her sister in her illness and developed certain coping patterns that relied on Karen's support. When Karen's kidneys failed, her family could not accept it. She told me:

Mother can't listen to *my* problems—I start talking and she always interrupts me to talk about her *own* problems. She doesn't want to hear about my illness. Because my sister was *really sick*, my mother always told me when I was growing up—how thankful I should be because I had my health. She said that I shouldn't complain and all, that I should keep it all inside. She really has this thing about doctors and hospitals—just doesn't want any part of it.

Her mother never visited her while she was on dialysis and rarely talked to her about her illness. Her father, on the other hand, did not understand or attempt to learn about his diabetes and had quite a lot of trouble with his illness. "He doesn't manage too well so he asks me what to do and I tell him about his medication and his diet and so on." Karen said that her family did not know what to do with her.

Karen approached the dialysis staff, expressing a desire for a kidney transplant. Although this procedure is generally contraindicated for patients with severe, underlying diabetes, the physician in the unit did not tell her that a transplant would be impossible. However, the staff suggested that finding a related living donor would be the only possible condition in which they would consider the procedure. The three family members living with her were ruled out, so Karen called her brother to tell him of this possibility. A staff member from the dialysis unit also talked with him about what it would mean to be a kidney donor. Her brother said that he could not come for the necessary tests (for histocompatibility), but if the staff could arrange for him to have the tests done where he lived and mailed, he would do it. He never had the tests taken, however, and her hopes for a transplant were dashed. She did not get "the gift" from her brother. She called her brother "forgetful." Often, in passing, with a shrug of her shoulders, she would say that "maybe I'll get a transplant from my brother. I don't know. . . ."

Outside of the hospital, Karen centered her social life on her son, who was four years old. She would talk of him constantly and, with a tremendous sense of parental pride, recount his exploits at nursery school, his extensive imagination and his intelligence. He was clearly a source of joy in her life, but he was also a major responsibility that, at times, she found difficult to manage. He spent his day in a day-care center near their apartment from Monday to Friday, and stayed with

Karen's mother during her Saturday morning dialysis sessions (she is on a Tuesday–Thursday–Saturday schedule, 8:00 A.M.–2:00 P.M. Most days when he arrived home she was extremely tired, but she tried her best to be an active playmate for her son. She was very concerned about his future, specifically his education. She did not want to send him to a neighborhood inner-city school ("They don't teach them anything there"), and hoped to enroll him in a private school the following year. This would be quite an expense for her, as the school she wanted him to attend charged a tuition of $1,800 a year. Karen rarely mentioned the boy's father, only to say that her son sometimes visited him. She was never married to him and did not talk about that experience.

Before the onset of her kidney disease, Karen had been employed as a night clerk in the police department. She worked nights because she was enrolled full time in a local community college, studying social work. She continued to work during the first stages of her illness and took a leave of absence when her worsening condition forced her to be treated on an in-patient basis. After her kidneys failed, she attempted to return to her job. However, the late hours and the strain of maintenance dialysis resulted in her finally quitting her job. (She had fallen asleep at her desk on a number of occasions.) She continued with her schooling but switched to a part-time schedule.

With no source of income, Karen finally became a public aid recipient. This changed her life dramatically over a two-year period, as she went from a working college student, with aspirations to a career as a social worker, to a welfare recipient. The situation sorely rubbed against her independent spirit and her pride. She finally moved into a public housing project because she could not keep up with the rent payments on her old apartment. Welfare provided a homemaker to come in two times a week to help her with household chores. She found this beneficial but had trouble adapting to her new apartment, which, she said, "is too small, but I don't have the money to get anything larger . . . right away."

Karen became unable to cope with the stress of college classes. When she first talked about her educational goals, she expressed a strong interest in becoming a medical social worker. Soon after she was forced to quit her job, however, school also became a problem. Without a car, she would take a cab to class, which was quite a distance from her apartment. Soon she felt too tired to get to both of her classes, and she dropped one. She said that she would take it again next semester when she thought that she would be feeling stronger. Her enthusiasm at this point was apparently only slightly diminished, and she still talked in definite terms of eventually finishing—though she knew that it would now be more difficult and would probably take longer. By the end of two more months Karen had missed so many sessions of her one remaining class that she had to speak to a counselor to explain her problems. She was afraid that she would lose her financial assistance because she was not keeping up the required hours. Karen also was concerned that the professor would think that she could not do the work: "I can do the work, it's not that hard—I just get so tired going there after the hospital and all." Her strong sense of self-determination made it difficult for her to accept the possibility that she was physically unable to take the class, even though she really wanted to complete it.

Finally her will broke down. "I just don't have the energy—the *motivation* to do this school thing—I feel too tired." After this point, she never mentioned again her career goals or any thoughts of working at a regular job. She thought that she might take up typing in her home, but she did not seem excited about that prospect. The incremental but nearly complete demise of her educational plans combined with a parallel loss of control over her living and financial situation represents the staggering impact of this disease on her life experience. She continued to be a devoted parent to her son, directing her energies to helping him. Karen hoped that his future would be bright and prayed that she would be a part of it.

Chronic Disease—The Reciprocal Nature of its Impact

As can be surmised from these two case histories, it would be fairly limiting to speak of the impact of this disease *on* (in a unilineal sense) the individual's life experience. The situation is better described as an interactive resonation between disease condition and the psychosocial matrix of the persons involved. As such, treatment staff, social support groups (families, friends), and economic systems all play a part in structuring the illness experience. In the case of ESRD, this is both an intensely personal and a shared experience. It differs qualitatively from acute, episodic illness and is not merely the serial summation of illness events. In the case of ESRD, to a greater extent than with most diseases, patients' attitudes and behaviors affect the course if not the direction of the disease process; patients' actions in such day-to-day functions as eating and drinking are critically important. Treatment staff are acutely aware of the patient-as-partner aspect of this condition and attempt, through various means, to ensure the best possible "fit" between patient behaviors and therapeutic imperatives. A "good fit" most often results in a generally positive staff attitude toward the patient, and although it cannot ensure a better course of the disease or prolong the life of the individual, this situation avoids much dissonance between patient and staff that can influence the illness experience. (However, the existential aspects of the illness for the patients can still be acute and even be exacerbated by attempts to maintain the fit and by the overt "rewards" for this behavior in the face of internal conflicts.) A "poor fit" can result in a high degree of tension between treatment staff and the patient, in limited trust between them, and in mutually negative categorizations (patient labeled "difficult," "a problem patient," "immature"; staff labeled "unresponsive," "pushy," or "stupid"). This situation generates a considerable degree of psychosocial dissonance between staff and patient and, more often than not, tends to exaggerate episodic treatment problems into "crises" with concomitant admonitions and blame. The experience becomes one of struggle and competition rather than concordance and understanding. (It is not entirely clear that this struggle—on the patient's part—is as negative a condition as it is often considered. This is to say, there might be a secondary gain from this behavior in terms of emotional survival.)

With this as a very general framework in which to view the impact of illness, let me return to the two cases. Karen seems to fall into the latter category—the poor fit. She was called a difficult patient, a problem. Karen was admonished about her management of her diabetic condition, which has resulted in occasional increases in her glucose level. I observed numerous interactions when Karen was confronted by a staff person who expressed strong dissatisfaction about her self-care of the diabetes. This made Karen feel guilty and fearful, and she would attempt an explanation for her condition. On the occasions when I was present, the staff person involved seemed not to have the time or patience for explanations—the "numbers" told enough. It is understood that the staff, in such an intense treatment setting, is also under duress; my point is not to pass moral judgment on any one staff member. What is important is the nature of the process, the repeated impact on Karen that influenced her negative attitude toward her experiences in the hospital and heightened her awareness and internalization of her label as "problem patient." She said to me, "They don't know what to do with me. . . . You know they [staff] really think that I'm difficult. . . . I fight with them. I always seem to be fighting with them."

Bill, on the other hand, was a good fit. He survived on the preferred method of treatment and exemplified the independence that the treatment staff hoped to inculcate in patients. Because he was self-employed, aggressive, and verbal, Bill was a model patient who was called on to give pep talks to patients, to meet with the media, and to talk at grand rounds. With a large and supportive family, and with support from his neighbors and community, Bill had the foundation to become an "exceptional" patient.

In the treatment of ESRD, today's exceptional patients will become a problem at some later time. The trajectory moves one way— toward increasing complications, frustration, and death. It is easy to support those patients who display the courage to survive *and* are successful. Would it not be better to recognize the courage it takes to maintain the will to survive under less exceptional circumstances?

Technical Promise and Treatment Realities

In the last three chapters I have tried to illustrate the multiple issues surrounding the social construction of a catastrophic disease. Two contrasting models of ESRD have been described, one primarily rooted in clinical science and professional interests, the other based on day-to-day struggles with the illness experience. Perhaps the most interesting question that follows from this juxtaposition of medical technology and experience is why this highly unstable and inherently contradictory "reality"—ESRD treatment—does not fall apart, why it functions as well as it does.

The clinical model influences the phenomenology of illness experience, but the categorization of problems and definition of solutions that derive from medical knowledge break down continually in practice. Patients and staff both experience a sensation of drowning in a sea of conflicting information and uncertain purpose. Yet the thin thread of "tentative certainty" offered by the clinical framework weaves this apparently dysfunctional treatment culture together and keeps it afloat. Patients and members of the treatment staff face together the problem of how to establish social relations in the context of treatment. It is important to recognize that this technologically oriented model offers false promises to both staff persons and patients. However, patients and staff both rebel against and also embrace the clinical model in an attempt to develop a collective strategy for coping.

To the treatment staff, the clinical construction of ESRD presents two techniques, dialysis and transplantation, that are difficult and require highly skilled practitioners. As the descriptions of patient-staff dynamics have shown, the acquisition of technical skill in treating ESRD is not sufficient to provide for successful patient outcomes, whether envisioned in terms of years of survival or quality of surviving life. There are just too many important social aspects of ESRD care that the clinically derived treatment model fails to or is unable to incorporate. When members of the treatment staff are continually faced with unexpected patient deaths for reasons beyond their understanding and expertise, they can become confused or depressed and react in a number of ways. Staff members will quit the ESRD unit and transfer to a different part of the hospital, usually one in which patient care seems more predictable and controllable, as in a general medicine floor. The staff turnover rate is quite high in many renal units. Others will remain in the ESRD unit and develop coping strategies for themselves such as the joking responses to uncertainty. Such responses and the related uses of gallows humor are characteristic of unstable social relationships.[2] The transcripts of the staff meetings indicate that there is a high degree of residual tension surrounding most treatment decisions. In some cases staff anxieties are focused on a particular problem patient so that staff-patient conflict arises, usually with a detrimental effect on the patient.

The promise of survival, with some measure of personal dignity, that dialysis and transplantation appear to offer is not always fulfilled. Many ESRD patients undergo continual struggles both with the hospital staff and with their disease. Those patients who are able to survive with dignity seem to do so through the force of their personality, tremendous inner strength, and broad networks of social and economic support. But a strong patient may have to overcome intense opposition from members of the treatment staff, who are challenged by patients who have "a mind of their own."

Both patients and practitioners are constrained by the "rules" of the ESRD treatment drama—a set of technological presuppositions about the manner in which the problems of chronic illness should be addressed. But there is considerable asymmetry in the distribution of social costs in the clinical construction of ESRD. Although patients and staff both take part in a contradictory social process, their stakes are quite different. Care providers can become depressed and can lose the desire to practice this profession. Patients, on the other hand, can lose the will to live, experience a protracted, technically mediated death, and become the center of a network of stressful social pressures affecting family and friends.

The staff tends to minimize the social impact of the disease and attempts to limit the problem of illness to a technical definition. They impose an artificial sense of certainty with a very important consequence for the quality of care. Their doing so removes the problem of ESRD as expressed by the patients to the margins of "professional" problem definition.

Generally, the patient account speaks to a social crisis. The loss of a job or the reverberating effects on family and on the quality of social life are typical and problems patients consider as central in their illness experience. Within the patient account, survival with dignity and not survival at any cost becomes a definition of the effectiveness of treatment. The stress that results from the imposition of certainty by the clinical account, the narrowing of the acceptable range of illness-related problems, creates additional problems for the ESRD patient. Patients must struggle, often with heroic efforts, to achieve recognition of the social nature of their illness experience. They do not understand why much more effort is not directed toward problems within this broader context.

The Impact of Patient and Clinical Accounts on Public Policy Formation

The problems associated with the treatment of ESRD are characteristic of catastrophic illnesses. To begin with, the clinical and the patient accounts provide radically different definitions of what constitutes the core problem.[3] Clinical accounts generally label diseases within a pathophysiological framework. They approach problem solving from a technical perspective—that is, problems are thought of, in a sense, as puzzle solving—and they attempt, at least implicitly, to limit uncertainty by placing more complex effects, such as social and quality aspects of treatment, at the margins of clinical discourse. The patient account, however, emphasizes the social context of the medical crisis. It draws attention to the fact that the crisis is a different experience for patients from different classes and age groups; it considers survival with dignity and not survival at any biologic cost as a standard for the effectiveness of treatment; and, finally, it reflects the stress caused by the imposition of clinical certainty on the uncertain social problems of ESRD.

In most general terms, I would suggest the following model to understand how these very different accounts are negotiated as public policy regarding ESRD is formed. Such policy making must define what constitutes the problem of chronic illness and long-term care. Patients and health providers enter the treatment context with very different historical backgrounds, which influence how they will experience this shared context of the clinic. Patients bring into the clinic their historical social conditions. When these two groups come together within the shared social space of the clinic, the patients' illness experience and the practitioners' medical uncertainty interact. This interaction suggests that problems in illness experience represent the flip side of practitioners' perceived problems with medical uncertainty. Both groups express the same ambiguity within the clinical setting, an ambiguity that is emphasized by the fact that the chronic disease being treated is itself ambiguous.

Figure 1 suggests how this complex web of experience, consisting of the illness of patients and the uncertainty of practitioners, forms. Each presents a source of information to provide an account of the problem from which a dominant account of the problem arises. In Figure 2, the dotted line from illness experience to the dominant account represents the fact that patient input to the definition of the clinical problem is far less than the medical input. The patient's perspective of the problem is underrepresented and the clinical input into the dominant account is disproportionately emphasized.

Figure 1
The Interaction of the Illness Experience and Medical Uncertainty

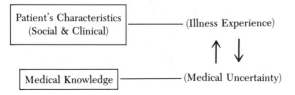

Figure 2
Constructing a Dominant Account

(Illness Experience) . . . .   "Dominant Account"

↑ ↓

(Medical Uncertainty)   1. Maximum Certainty
                             2. Reconstruct Illness Experience

                                      ↓

                                  (Policy)

The dominant account of ESRD (and I suggest this is the same for other ambiguous chronic diseases) characteristically emphasizes the maximum amount of clinical certainty that can be expressed about the course and treatment of this condition. Simultaneously, it reconstructs the uncertainty that is so much a part of experience into a framework that is less threatening to clinical practice and to the public perception of the effectiveness of technology. This dominant account, in fact, becomes the public policy definition of the problem.

In Figure 3, I have combined these two parts of the process. This model attempts to portray the relationships among patient characteristics, illness experience, medical knowledge, and medical uncertainty as differential influences on the way we tend to see a problem such as ESRD public policy.

In ESRD and, by analogy, in other uncertain chronic diseases involving life extending technologies, a few issues seem to be particularly important. Policy concerning the uncertainty of technologically extended lives seems to be influenced by accounts of the illness problem that are overdetermined by the clinical perspective and that see solutions to those problems in terms of either federal payment for expensive technologies or the creation of a private market to provide

Figure 3
Synthesis of Figures 1 and 2

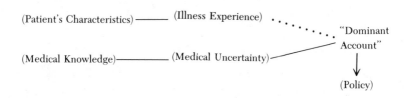

(Patient's Characteristics) ——— (Illness Experience) . . .
                                                          . . . . "Dominant
                                                               Account"
(Medical Knowledge)——————— (Medical Uncertainty)

                                                               ↓

                                                           (Policy)

services more effectively. These approaches address the parts of the problem that emphasize specific defects and their treatment but ignore the broader social context. Rarely addressed in public policy forums and in today's political milieu are the effects that social variables and complicating factors such as patients' class and economic status have on the chronic illness experience. Therefore, it is not surprising that such variables as quality of care are not usually discussed. Such problems as family stress, job stress, and the community effects of illness are all the more difficult to consider in shaping a public approach to solving these health problems, especially in federal legislation.

There are two major problems. First, because the clinical account is so intricately linked with the definition of problems that have their solutions in expensive medical technologies and because the results of treatment fall so short of the technical promise, patients, providers, and policy makers are all left to deal with residual problems, and all are unsatisfied with the solutions that are proposed for the treatment of uncertain diseases. Programs such as the federal program for renal disease patients are expensive to the federal government and stressful to patients and staff.

Second, this tendency to use the dominant account of chronic illness to develop public policies reinforces a system of technological fixes and social control that tends to exacerbate the problems that it ostensibly addresses. It only makes more difficult the public task of providing for humane treatment or preventing chronic illness, a subject I will consider in Part II.

PART II

Federal Policy and the
Social Context of
Mortality
Can You Get There from Here?

In 1973, ESRD became the first catastrophic illness for which the federal government would pay treatment costs (through Medicare) for nearly all persons, both under and over the age of sixty-five. It remains the only illness so subsidized. Over 70,000 persons are now being treated in this program; the different treatments used include hemodialysis, peritoneal dialysis, and transplantation, and they are offered in a variety of settings: hospitals, free-standing facilities, home. As I discussed in Part I, these treatments do not cure the condition; they prolong life for varying lengths of time, depending on a variety of clinical, sociodemographic, and social factors.[1]

Federal policy makers must consider the following interrelated problems: the escalating costs of ESRD treatment, whether or not ESRD patients become "rehabilitated," whether or not cost-effective treatments are used to the extent possible, and, finally, whether or not treatment facilities provide efficient care. These are extremely complex issues that are deeply embedded in the nuances of patient care. To make such judgments one must have, at minimum, comprehensive data on the mortality and morbidity associated with ESRD.[2]

The Health Care Financing Administration (HCFA), which manages this program within the Department of Health and Human Services, collects such data through the ESRD Medical Information System (MIS) for each treatment facility. Reporting completeness, however, ranges from a low of 20 percent to a high of 70 percent of patients.[3] Developing reasonable and effective program policies demands an understanding of the causes of poor survival. Survival might seem simple enough to measure: when does a patient die? It might also seem straightforward to determine what the patient died from. Here I address the issue of cause of death in a treated ESRD population. My particular concern is whether the federal data accurately represent the social context of mortality in this important chronic illness, rather than reflecting only proximate clinical correlates. Is there a social matrix of dying in ESRD which, if understood, could provide the information needed for better quality of care?

The patients I studied included all ESRD patients treated at a large New England teaching hospital who died between 1973 and 1978 (N = 50). Those for whom complete medical records could not be found were excluded from the sample, leaving a sample size of 40 with substantial social and demographic variation. The age range of patients at the time of death was 23–76, with a mean of 48.

The 40 medical records were carefully reviewed by a panel of trained outside reviewers: a physician, a nurse, a social worker, and an epidemiologist. An explicit protocol was developed for chart review to assess the cause of death, incorporating the autopsy report and a careful retrospective analysis of social and behavioral factors in patient care preceding death. Data were classified by a consensus judgment of the panel. The reviewers were not allowed to see the cause of death reported to the government. The cause of death for each case was assigned by reviewers as instructed by the ESRD death notification form. This form lists sixteen disease-oriented and five social context-oriented classifications for cause of death. Social and contextual factors can also be accommodated by an "other" category and further defined in a "remarks" section of the form.

Reviewers' classifications were then compared with the reports of primary cause of death reported to the government. The reporting form that assigns death to a specific cause is completed by one of the staff nephrologists. The study unit's rate of compliance in filing these reports was 100 percent; there were no patients in the sample for whom a comparative cause was not available.

The frequencies of causes of death reported on the death notification form are presented in Table 8, column 1. The distribution of causes found on the reports is consistent with the national profile of ESRD causes of death reported from many other programs. Cardiac-

Table 8

Reclassifications of Reported Cause of Death
in 40 ESRD Cases

Cause of Death	Death Notification Form	Chart Review
Cardiac-related	24	7
Cerebrovascular	2	3
Septicemia	2	3
Respiratory arrest	2	0
Chronic renal failure	2	0
Embolism (air)	1	0
Embolism (pulmonary)	1	0
Infection (pulmonary)	0	1
Infection (other)	1	1
Pancreatitis	0	1
Malignancy	1	2
Accidental treatment-related	1	7
Formal withdrawal from dialysis	0	2
Other		
Dietary indiscretion	0	11
Suicide	0	1
Euthanasia	0	1
Unknown	3	0
Total	40	40

Source: Alonzo L. Plough and S. R. Salem, "Social and Contextual Factors in the Analysis of Mortality in End-Stage Renal Disease Patients," *American Journal of Public Health* 72 (1982), pp. 1293–95.

related causes are the number-one category of death listed, representing over 50 percent of the sample. The analysis of the medical records by the reviewer panel, focusing particularly on the period immediately preceding the death of the patient, resulted in a different assessment of the causes of death (Table 8, column 2). Dietary indiscretions were the primary underlying cause of death, representing 27 percent of the reclassified deaths. "Dietary indiscretions" was a category that represented charted indications of severe problems with dietary compliance immediately preceding the death of a patient. Examples included consumption of large quantities of restricted foods (potato chips and beer) and disregard for the fluid restrictions of an ESRD patient's diet.

Accidental death related to treatment represented 17 percent of the reclassified deaths in this sample. This category consists of deaths related to problems with technical aspects of dialysis treatment and, in the opinion of the review panel, the deaths were preventable. On a case-by-case basis, agreement as to cause of death occurred in only 25 percent of the 40 cases; in 75 percent, the cause of death reported by the panel review differed from that on the HCFA form.

Divergent judgments were found across all causes, but the only category of deaths large enough to examine further were those attributed to cardiac-related causes (Table 9). The panel felt that of these 24 deaths (60 percent of the sample), 13 (52 percent) resulted from factors directly related to the treatment of ESRD (dietary indiscretion, 8; treatment-related accidents, 5). Only five of the initial reports were unchanged by the panel of reviewers.

Much of the difference between the federal data reports and the panel judgments can be attributed to the difficulty of representing the context (i.e., treatment and psychosocial factors) as well as the immediate clinical cause of death on the federal form. The review panel's independent and multiprofessional character may also represent a different perspective on the allocation of a death to a particular cause than that of a physician associated with the unit. Factors such as

Table 9
Reclassifications of Reported Cardiac Deaths
in 24 ESRD Cases

Revised Cause of Death	Absolute Frequency
Dietary indiscretion	8
Treatment-related accidents	5
Cardiac-related deaths	5
Pulmonary infection	1
Septicemia	1
Infection, other	1
Pancreatitis	1
Formal withdrawal from dialysis	1
Suicide	1
Total	24

Source: Alonzo L. Plough and S. R. Salem, "Social and Contextual Factors in the Analysis of Mortality in End-Stage Renal Disease Patients, *American Journal of Public Health* 72 (1982), pp. 1293–95.

dietary indiscretion and treatment-related accidents are intricately woven into the social process and content of ESRD treatment and not easily determined without a careful retrospective review of the medical record.[4] Although cardiac arrest was clearly the proximate clinical event to the death of many of the patients in this sample, the social and contextual conditions surrounding mortality in this population of ESRD patients points to a more complex issue than is indicated by the term *cardiac arrest.*

It is through this type of selective medical accounting that the clinical framework is transformed into a *bureaucratic* account of the problem of survival in ESRD. Even in the case of a supposedly easy-to-document event, death, the social context of treatment is the key. Only through an understanding of the dynamics of experience in ESRD treatment can the clinical label *cardiac death* be reconstructed into the more meaningful category of *dietary indiscretion.*

Even this reconstruction is only a starting point for a more thorough social phenomenology of death in the ESRD clinic. Clearly, as we have seen, the problem is more than an episode of noncompliance, giving in, giving up, suicide, or any other simplistic labeling of a patient as individually deficient. The dietary regimen is quite difficult and demanding, and patients can reasonably decide when they have had enough. Also, dietary indiscretion could be an indicator of a broader disenchantment with ESRD treatment. Such behavior might signal that from the patient's perspective the costs had begun to far exceed the benefits of treatment.

On the other hand, this finding could have important implications for both ESRD patients and for future policy decisions. Perhaps an early intervention and preventive strategy to lower mortality in this population is possible. More aggressive efforts in patient education and staff awareness could create a more flexible environment for compliance with dietary restrictions. An increase in staff monitoring of patients who are undergoing center dialysis might reduce the number of treatment-related accidents. Changes in the death notification form to facilitate the reporting of social and contextual factors also seem to be indicated.

Future policy decisions are obviously affected when the data do not accurately depict a situation comprehensively. No reporting form can capture the dynamics of experience in ESRD, but it is especially important to at least understand what proportion of deaths are potentially preventable through direct intervention. Data systems that report clinical events in isolation fail to take into account the psychosocial and behavioral complexities surrounding the terminal event.

This is but one example of how broad ranges of issues in ESRD are narrowed to better fit the limitations of the viewers' paradigm. The federal policy developed for ESRD can be characterized by such selective accounting of problems, whether the issue is costs, quality, the role of the market, or the meaning of death.

CHAPTER FIVE

Regulating Medical Uncertainty

Many of the problems of ESRD are the problems of chronic disease in general, which poses diverse health policy issues. Chronic or long-term illnesses range from long-term restrictive conditions such as arthritis to debilitating systemic diseases such as diabetes, hypertension, and cancer. The magnitude of the chronic illness problem is reflected in the estimate that 50 percent of the national population, excluding residents in institutions, have some type of chronic condition.[1] The chronic disease category also includes illnesses that are suddenly fatal. Chronic diseases are often termed "catastrophic" because of the radical impact that they have on the quality and duration of life. Treatments for these conditions are quite costly and are responsible for 40 percent of total health care costs.[2] The social and political ramifications of this type of illness are far-reaching, extending beyond the context of medical treatment. The complex network of issues that surround chronic disease involve (as we have seen) the patient, the family, the medical treatment team, and public policy makers as they attempt to allocate resources for the treatment of these diseases.

Chronic kidney failure is a good example of a chronic disease for a variety of reasons. It fits our definition of a catastrophic illness. There are two costly treatment methods—dialysis and transplantation—without which a person with ESRD will not live. These treatments, however, do not cure this condition. They offer a prolongation of life, the duration of which depends on a variety of factors, both treatment related and social-psychological. Of particular interest is that chronic kidney failure is the only catastrophic illness for which the federal government pays treatment costs for nearly all persons. As a result of the decision to provide public funds to support this treatment system, the government has monitored participating ESRD treatment programs to provide data for future policies and regulations. These, in turn, will directly affect the system of health care services.[3] From a national health policy perspective, there has been concern about the efficiency of ESRD treatment in the light of its cost—reaching 1.7 billion per year in 1983.[4] The federal government has attempted to control the escalating costs of delivering services to ESRD patients by legislation and regulations designed to slow the rate of program growth. The primary thrust of cost-control efforts has been to promote so-called cost-effective modes of treatments and to influence the distribution of patients among alternative modalities. Regulating cost-effective ESRD care has proven to be a highly complex and difficult task. It involves both an ongoing assessment of the use of alternative renal technologies and the development of strategies to control costs and maintain the quality of delivered services.

In this discussion of the development of federal policy for ESRD and of its impact on the organization of ESRD services, I will focus on the assumptions of federal policy that provided the opportunity for private markets in equipment and services to develop between 1972 and 1980. The implications for ESRD patients of this partnership of the public and private sectors and its impact on the dynamics of care will be considered. The problem of constructing a public policy for the delivery of services to a population suffering a chronic disease for which there is substantial ambiguity regarding appropriate treatment is the central issue for the next three chapters. I will discuss serious problems that have emerged in the regulation of ESRD treatment: the nationalization of clinical uncertainty, the canonization of halfway technologies, and the dubious assumptions regarding the for-profit sector's ability to balance cost control with quality of care as it provides public services for chronic illness.

Federal Activities and ESRD

The clinical complexity of ESRD, as discussed in Chapter 1, is related to questions about the relative effectiveness of the various modes of treatment. Medical treatment of kidney failure was in a relatively early stage of development before 1972. Generally accepted standards for clinical intervention were not available. Dialysis and transplantation moved from the experimental to the therapeutic category, but not through an explicit assessment such as a randomized clinical trial.[5] From the perspective of clinicians and their successful patients, the adequacy of treatment was not an issue. Dialysis and transplantation provided an extension of life where none had previously been available. The simple dichotomy of life versus death presented a strong rhetorical framework that gave momentum to a moral definition of the problem—the absence of treatment for any ESRD patient could not be considered ethical. Public opinion demanded federal intervention to ensure that access to treatment would be independent of ability to pay for these expensive therapies.[6] Federal policy regarding ESRD developed within a highly charged environment where a policy to deliver services preceded an assessment of the appropriate use of ESRD technology.

Federally initiated program analysis before 1972 consisted of two long reports, both of which appeared in 1967. The Public Health Service submitted a report to the surgeon general, *Kidney Disease Program Analysis*. This report by Dr. Benjamin Burton discussed and evaluated the extent of federal research effort related to all forms of kidney disease. The so-called Burton Report was the first comprehensive analysis of data on renal disease morbidity and mortality. It cited a death rate of 60,000 persons a year and a prevalence of 8 million people who suffered from kidney disease. By focusing on the effects of renal disease on the economy, the Burton Report emphasized cost considerations that were to play a prominent role in subsequent legislative efforts.

These patients experienced approximately 50 million days of restricted activity, 64 million days of bed disability, and almost 16 million lost workdays. The costs of these illnesses amounted to $1,210 million, making kidney disease the fifth most costly disease in the nation. Further, it is estimated that some 3,300,000 people have an unrecognized and undiagnosed infection of the kidney.[7]

This report suggested a range of possible government interventions, from a minimal $15 million a year for research and training to an all-out, comprehensive treatment program estimated (as of 1971) to cost $200 million a year. No specific recommendations were advanced in this document. Furthermore, this report gave only a tentative endorsement to dialysis and transplantation.

Three months later the Bureau of the Budget created a committee to review the policy problems posed by chronic kidney disease. Chaired by Dr. C. W. Gottschalk, the committee suggested "a national treatment program aimed at providing chronic dialysis or transplantation for all of the American population for whom it is medically indicated."[8] Its report strongly asserted that the two main treatment modalities were sufficiently well advanced to warrant being therapeutically applied in a national program.

The Gottschalk Report became the study that did most to determine federal policy decisions regarding ESRD. It provided the basic rationale for subsequent legislation. A few of its other major points included:

1. Resources are limited and cause tragic choices to be made.
2. Federal assistance is mandatory to provide treatment for all.
3. A commitment must be made to provide money for research on more efficient machines.
4. Transplants have been demonstrated to be cost effective.
5. Cadavers are the most appropriate source of kidneys for transplants.
6. Funding should come from Title XVIII of the Social Security Act.

These six guidelines become very important in the future development of the federal role in ESRD.

Legislation

The categorical health programs of the 89th Congress (Heart Disease, the Cancer and Stroke Act, the Regional Medical Program, and Comprehensive Health Planning) had set the stage for disease-specific federal interventions in U.S. health policy. The rapid growth of the National Institutes of Health (NIH) during the 1950s and 1960s firmly established the federal government's prominent role in basic medical research and, to a lesser extent, program development. The general model was one of categorically funded research and demonstration projects based in medical centers. The dominant policy position vis-à-vis the *politically* visible chronic diseases was to develop programs combining basic research and high technology. Demonstrations were conducted to evaluate the effectiveness of the products of this research. The general delivery of services and their attendant costs were implicitly left to the private, fee-for-service market, with the exception of two groups: the poor (Medicaid) and the old (Medicare). Such was the policy structure within which the more comprehensive federal approach to ESRD developed.

A primary concern of the early advocates for a federal program for ESRD was to establish that a cost-effective technology *was* available and that such treatment would have a rehabilitative impact—returning persons who were stricken with ESRD to economic productivity. Congressional hearings emphasized the devastating personal and social costs of ESRD. Congressmen who had personal experiences with ESRD patients presented compelling statements to that effect.[9]

Estimates of the potential demand for ESRD services were artificially low, based upon then-current criteria regarding medical suitability for treatment. During the late 1960s, any patient with systemic disease (e.g., diabetes, cancer, or vascular disease) or over age fifty-five was not considered suitable for dialysis or transplant. (With the further availability of federal monies, this situation would change, a partial explanation of the "unexpected cost" phenomenon.)

Finally, during the 92nd Congress (1972) and after only four minutes of floor debate, an amendment to the Social Security Act was passed and became law on October 30, 1972 (P.L. 92-603). The "kidney amendment" (Section 299 Id) provided, for the first time, that a federal program would have responsibility to reimburse nearly all costs (80 percent) for virtually all persons with a particular diagnosis.

The Congress amended Title XVIII of the Social Security Act (Medicare) to provide full Medicare coverage for at least six months to all individuals, regardless of age, who were diagnosed as having ESRD. In general, Part A of Medicare covers in-patient hospital costs of dialysis and kidney transplantation and Part B covers physician services, out-patient hospital services, and other out-of-hospital medical services and supplies. As a result, more than 90 percent of the country's population suffering from this disease now have sufficient financial protection to pay for most available medical care. Renal disease is still the only illness for which Medicare pays the treatment costs for almost all persons.

Significantly, the 1972 amendments provided a unique regulatory authority for the health area by authorizing the secretary of the Department of Health, Education, and Welfare to establish standards of minimal utilization rates and medical review boards to assure appropriateness of care, and to reimburse only those facilities that met such standards. This created an unprecedented capacity for governmental intervention into the details of standards for practice in medical care. [10]

The uniqueness of this section of the 1972 law can be appreciated if one reflects on the fact that in the original 1963 Medicare amendments the Congress emphatically specified that no component of the Medicare program should infringe on the practice of medicine. Medicare was simply to be a funding mechanism to provide reimbursement for all approved services by all "authorized providers" and participating institutions. Federal standards for ESRD care go far beyond PSRO-type utilization measures and impinge on central elements of physician decision making such as choice of therapy.

Section 2991 was incorporated into the Social Security amendments as a floor amendment. In proposing the amendment on 30 September, Senator Vance Hartke projected that the cost of the program would be $250 million at the end of four years (1 July 1977) and that the first full year would cost the federal government $75 million.

The problem inherent in the implementation of the ESRD program began thirty days later with the signing of P. L. 92-603. The cost of planning for the program had been underestimated by almost 100 percent. By 1975 it became evident to a number of congressmen that the costs for the treatment were much higher than early estimates had indicated. The ESRD program under Medicare was reviewed in 1975 by the Subcommittee on Oversight of the House Ways and Means Committee. Just before the hearings, the Government Accounting Office (GAO) issued a report on the costs of their program. Both of these reports were highly critical of efforts to contain the costs of ESRD treatment and were

> deeply concerned with these high costs which place a heavy burden on the trust funds and general revenues. These costs also limit options to provide protection for the costs of treating equally deserving patients confronted with other forms of catastrophic disease such as hemophilia, stroke, cerebral palsy, cancer, and so forth. The committee seeks to insure that the costs of this program are limited to the absolute minimum while providing quality medical care to meet legitimate patient needs. [11]

The charge from the Congress, carried through to the most recent attempts to change the renal legislation, is to maintain access and quality in the ESRD program but also to control costs to the extent possible under those constraints. Cost, however, remains a critical problem, and the form of federal interventions has added to the cost problem.

Paying for ESRD Services

The 1972 amendment permitted DHEW to limit the number of providers who would be reimbursed for dialysis treatment to those who would accept a new system of practitioner reimbursement (not fee-for-service as with other physicians' services paid for under Part B), and to limit strictly the number of hospitals that could be reimbursed to those performing a minimum number of transplants each year. In essence, the physicians who provided dialysis treatments were the first group of American physicians to be put on a national fee schedule. Traditionally, Medicare has reimbursed physicians on the basis of "reasonable charges" under Part B. Since virtually all maintenance dialysis patients are eligible for Medicare benefits, Medicare pays for nearly all dialysis services. As a consequence, there was little or no valid non-Medicare data to determine what the "prevailing" charges are. How could a private market set the rate when no private market existed?

On the other hand, dialysis is a medical therapy that can be viewed as a rather standard "machine-run" procedure for which definable cost can be estimated. Initially, DHEW attempted to include physician payments as a part of the facility cost per dialysis rather than reimburse it as a separate charge. Because physician's services are not needed at each dialysis session, but only as emergency backup or for general supervision, this approach seemed warranted. Ultimately, policies retreated from this position and established a "comprehensive reimbursement" method calculated to produce an average physician charge of $200 per month for each dialysis patient under his or her supervision. The physician reimbursement system continues to be controversial.

The initial regulations offered the physicians caring for ESRD patients a choice between two alternative payment mechanisms. Under Method I, supervisory services provided by the physicians to dialysis patients are reimbursable to the facility since the facility is required to provide these services under the general supervision of a physician. Some of the reimbursable supervisory services include: being available for consultation with patients and staff; overseeing the performance of dialysis on individual patients; reviewing laboratory data; monitoring the patient's medical status, vital signs, and medications; authorizing supplies and medications and evaluating diet and psychosocial problems. Nonroutine services, such as handling life-threatening complications, were reimbursable to the physician by the third-party intermediary in accordance with the standard reasonable-charge criteria. Additionally, physician services provided to hospital ESRD patients for reasons other than maintenance dialysis and to home patients were also reimbursed according to the reasonable-charge criteria. This method could be employed in a free-standing facility only if all physicians associated with the unit agreed.

Alternatively, under Method II, physicians could elect to receive a comprehensive monthly payment from the third-party intermediary for their services to maintenance dialysis patients in a facility, at home, or in training for self-dialysis. The fee may be paid directly to the patient or to the physician if he or she accepts assignment. This method recognized the dialysis patient's need for continued management over long periods of time. It was also responsive to physicians' charging patterns for comparable services. HCFA issued guidelines that attempted to ensure that services for which remuneration was made were actually delivered. Those services not reimbursable through the monthly payment format were covered by the reasonable-charge criteria. Reimbursements for self-dialysis training was made to the physician upon the patient's completion of the training program and were in addition to any payments received under Methods I or II. This provided a financial incentive to the physician to keep the number of dropouts at a minimum.

Comprehensive payments were made for all the surgeon's services incurred in connection with renal transplantation, including pre- and postsurgical care, and immunosuppressant therapy for a period of sixty days. Payments for services incurred after this period were based on the reasonable-charge criteria.

Physician reimbursement policies can profoundly affect the distribution of patients in alternative treatment settings. The initial renal regulations encouraged the more costly utilization of in-center services under which payments were more easily handled, and physicians were able to use their time more efficiently by treating a large number of patients in the same center at the same time. In-center treatment was more cost-effective treatment for the physician. There also were economic disincentives to patients for at-home treatment; they had to pay for certain supplies. The original legislation had also motivated the patient to choose institutional treatment.[12]

Facility Payment

Excessive costs to the total system also derived from Medicare's policy for reimbursing facilities. Medicare recognized a maximum charge of $150 per treatment and reimbursed free-standing facilities at 30 percent of this charge. Hospital dialysis providers were reimbursed according to the Medicare cap or were reimbursed 80 percent of "allowable costs." As a result, reimbursable dialysis costs averaged something in excess of $19,000 in a free-standing facility and approximately $25,000 in a hospital-based facility. In part, the high fixed costs of administrative services and the broader range of services available in a hospital unit account for the higher unit costs. One estimate identified an average difference in costs of $58–$70 per procedure between dialysis in a free-standing facility and in a hospital.[13] Another source estimated an annual extra cost of $8,736 per patient for dialysis performed in a hospital. Very little was really known about dialysis costs, for the rapid growth of the federal program was a fast-moving target that made cost analyses almost impossible.

The Growth of Dialysis Centers

Few dialysis centers had existed before 1972, when the renal amendments added greatly to the demand for such services. By 1977 there were 895 approved facilities participating in the ESRD program. These facilities then provided 7,306 patient dialysis stations, served over 27,000 patients, and performed over 4 million treatments a year. As of 1 January 1977, 79.1 percent of the participating facilities were in the private sector and 20.9 percent were government supported. The ownership pattern is pictured in Figure 4.

There were dramatic and much-discussed increases in expenditures for ESRD from 1972 to 1978.[14] Costs rose much faster than was originally estimated. Table 10 presents the then current trends in Medicare costs. Cost projections varied widely, a problem that com-

Figure 4

Ownership of ESRD Dialysis Facilities, 1977

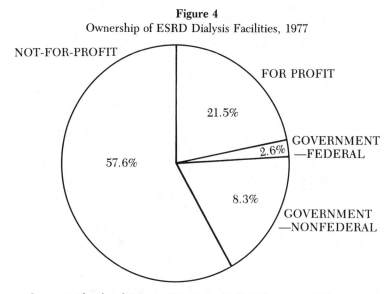

Source: A. Plough and R. Berry, "Regulating Medical Uncertainty: Policy Issues in End-Stage Renal Disease," in S. Altman and H. Sapalsky, eds., *Federal Health Programs* (Lexington, Mass.: Lexington Books, 1982).

plicated the development of policy. The reasons for increased costs were always unclear and controversial.

Two reasons seem to account for the increased expenditures for ESRD during the period. The first is the greater-than-expected utilization of dialysis services by patients who were suffering from other serious medical problems. Dialysis performed in a hospital presented minimal costs to the patient, and the hospital received reimbursement for all costs, including overhead. This influenced physicians to treat a much wider range of patients with dialysis, even though such a clinical intervention may have had marginal value in terms of survival. A second reason expenditures increased faster than expected was that patients, responding to an incentive in the legislation, switched from the less expensive (to the government) form of home dialysis to more costly treatment in a free-standing renal dialysis facility. This change in site increased the annual treatment costs per patient substantially, from about $15,000 to about $25,000. Before full Medicare coverage was available, some patients limited their personal costs by choosing home-based treatment. (Although

Table 10

Actual and Projected Costs for End-Stage Renal Disease, 1974–83

Fiscal Year	Total Costs to Medicare (millions of $)	Total National Costs (millions of $)	Patient Population
1974*	242.5	286.2	18,848
1975*	404.6	479.5	25,654
1976*	573.3	684.2	31,631
1977†	757.1	901.9	37,106
1978†	958.5	1,143.3	41,939
1979†	1,176.4	1,404.4	46,121
1980†	1,421.1	1,695.6	49,802
1981†	1,667.7	1,992.7	53,077
1982†	1,941.7	2,321.6	55,911
1983†	2,235.1	2,674.3	58,391

*Actual.
†Estimated.
Source: A. Plough and R. Berry, "Regulating Medical Uncertainty: Policy Issues in End-Stage Renal Disease," in S. Altman and H. Sapalsky, eds., *Federal Health Programs* (Lexington, Mass.: Lexington Books, 1982), p. 164.

some physicians are advocates of home treatments, many are not, for the social and psychological stress to patients and their families is considerable—see Chapters 2 and 3.)[15] Many patients, confronted by the financial disincentives (the normal $100 deductible and 25 percent co-insurance of Part B applied to home and free-standing facility dialysis but not to hospital dialysis, which was fully paid under Part A), switched to the more expensive form of in-center treatment.

The shift between modalities was quite significant from a cost perspective. The short-term costs of transplantation seem the lowest, home dialysis was considered the second least costly, and dialysis in a hospital or in a free-standing facility was considered the most costly treatment. Average annual costs of home dialysis and center dialysis ranged from $6,000 to over $22,760 and from $19,000 to $30,000, respectively. (Home treatment costs are substantially increased when the helper is paid.) First-year costs of transplantation are $20,000 to $25,000, with annual costs for physician services and immunosuppressive drug therapy of $2,000 to $3,000. Estimates vary from source to source, pointing again to the problem of the validation of costs for ESRD treatment. Table 11 presents some often-cited estimates of comparative costs.

Table 11
Comparative Costs in Various Alternative Treatment Settings

Source of Estimate	In-hospital		In-center		Home	
	$/Dialysis	$/Year	$/Dialysis	$/Year	$/Dialysis	$/Year
National Kidney Foundation	187	29,172	145	22,620	83	12,948
Social Administration	147	22,932	143	22,308	75	11,700*
Stange and Sumner	—	—	148	23,088	90	15,400†
Subcommittee on Health	—	—	183	29,000	38	6,000

Note: Annual costs are estimated on the basis of 156 treatments per year.
*Costs for year 1, including in-center training.
†Costs for following years.
Source: A. Plough and R. Berry, "Regulating Medical Uncertainty: Policy Issues in End-Stage Renal Disease," in S. Altman and H. Sapalsky, eds., *Federal Health Programs* (Lexington, Mass.: Lexington Books, 1982), p. 165.

The number of patients treated at home showed a decline from 39.8 percent in 1971 to 23.7 percent in 1976.[16] This precipitous decline elicited a revision of the renal amendments and a renewed attempt by HCFA to influence the dynamics of ESRD care delivery. Chasing program costs became the major activity of federal program officials.

Regulatory Responses—Policy Implementation

The magnitude of the cost problem in ESRD service delivery elicited continual changes in federal policies. The ESRD program had been conducted under interim regulations until the final regulations specifying the organizational and reimbursement structure of the ESRD program were published in late 1976, nearly five years after the program began. These regulations were further revised and amended by the HCFA to include mandatory reporting requirements for determination of reasonable charges for reimbursement, effective December 1977.

Federal regulations required ESRD facilities to form regional groups, or networks. The purpose of these networks was to coordinate federally funded programs to assure quality patient care at minimum costs. In order to be eligible for reimbursement, a dialysis unit must be a member of one of the thirty-two designated networks.[17] Although limited by geographic and population density differences, each established network serves a minimum of 3.5 million people. Additionally, each is required to have two renal transplantation centers, an organ procurement organization, histocompatibility testing capabilities, facilities for in-patient and chronic maintenance dialysis as well as programs for self-care dialysis training, and support services for home dialysis patients.

The networks are managed through a Coordinating Council, which acts as a liaison between the Bureau of Health Standards and Quality (BHSQ) and participating facilities. The BHSQ is charged with setting policies and guidelines for the Network Coordinating Councils, assessing the effectiveness of network operation, assisting the networks in developing an effective Medical Review system, and operating the ESRD Management Information System.

The impact of the renal networks on the goals of cost and quality control is, at the present time, unknown. Preliminary analysis indicates that there are conflicting and overlapping regulatory responsibilities between various state-level agencies such as the Health Systems Agencies (HSA) and state health planning agencies, who also have responsibility for ESRD planning. The networks do monitor dialysis center utilization requirements issued by HCFA's Bureau of Health Insurance but as yet have not established standards for quality assurance or a policy for proprietary dialysis care. In the bureaucratic rhetoric, it would be "discriminatory" to have special or restrictive policies toward the profit-making facilities.

To counter the rate of cost increases associated with the renal disease program, Congress passed an amendment to the renal amendment in 1978. Its principal thrust was to remove the economic disincentives for home dialysis and transplantations contained in the initial legislation. This law, P.L. 95-0292:

1. Waived the three-month waiting period for benefits if the patient elects a self-care program.
2. Supplied reimbursement coverge for disposable supplies required for home dialysis.
3. Supplied reimbursement coverage for periodic in-center supportive services.
4. Fully reimbursed ESRD facilities for equipment purchased for the exclusive use of home dialysis patients.
5. Provided for reimbursement of a paid assistant for home dialysis patients.

With these changes, the government hoped for an upward shift in the percentage of patients choosing home dialysis. This expectation was perhaps naive. The impact of regulatory change on the dynamics of patient flow in ESRD treatment seems complicated and quite resistant to federal tinkering.

Government reimbursement for ESRD treatment has had widespread ramifications. Among the most important has been the heightened interest in and the flow of people into the medical subspecialty of nephrology, and an increase in the treated ESRD population. In addition, there has been a significant shift to the apparently more expensive treatment settings such as in-hospital treatment. These have been the issues most extensively discussed in the current policy debate, over costs.

Another impact of this approach to legislation that has not been extensively analyzed is the development of the ESRD-related equipment industry and for-profit service providers. Governmental intervention in the marketplace has been the single most important factor influencing both supply and demand in these two sectors. It has been a boon to what was previously a small industry. As the single largest buyer of services, the government has had and will continue to have the greatest impact on the market's future.

Beyond the effect of the renal regulation the the private market, it can be argued that private industry has a potential impact on federal program goals. To gain some perspective on this important, reciprocal relation between regulation and the market, I will look in the next chapter at the two parts of the industry—proprietary dialysis facilities and manufacturing firms who produce and distribute supplies unique to ESRD treatment. Because of the major role that industrial research and development in supplies plays in establishing both the costs of treatment and the types of technologies available for use, an industry analysis may inform policy decision making.

I will examine the period immediately following the passage of the renal amendment and focus on the characteristics of the industry and the influence of federal funds on the growth of that industry. Then, I can consider the potential influence of the private sector itself on federal program costs.

CHAPTER SIX

The Market
Construction
of Disease

During the last few years there has been a growing debate concerning the role of the private, profit-making corporations in the delivery of health services. While this has become a central issue in health policy discussions at all levels, the evidence upon which both the proponents of the efficiency of free-market competition and the opponents of the medical-industrial complex argue the issue is slim. The policy dialogue on the corporate influence on health care in America is, in essence, a conflict of values and goals. Competing visions of the role of government, the limits of the profit motive, the right to health care, and the characteristics of an equitable society separate the various camps. Given the nature of this debate, ideology rather than evidence has driven current policy regarding the role of profit-making corporations in the health care system.

There is no more powerful ideology in America than the ideal of the free market and the sanctity of private enterprise. The application of the market metaphor to the health care system merely shifts the focus of these historically powerful cultural symbols to the treatment of disease. The ideology that opposes this symbolic incursion of the market into the system of health care is a far more diffuse and less powerful set of symbols. A fragile coalition consisting of consumer advocates, left and liberal health policy activists, and physicians concerned with the impact of the corporations on the independent practice of medicine wages an almost quixotic battle for justice, equity, and the primacy of patient needs over profits.

The momentum and the power now clearly reside with the advocates of market rationality. Federal health care policies in the United States have defined the most urgent problem as rising costs and the solution as cost containment through market-regulated competition. Other concerns such as quality of care or access to health care have taken a back seat to the implementation of a reimbursement strategy where Medicare sets in advance the rates it will pay for various services through the "diagnosis-related groups." This forms the cornerstone of the prospective payment system implemented in October 1983. As a result, the federal government has applied a model derived from the manufacturing-oriented discipline of operations research to the delivery of health services to sick people. The gamble is that the efficiencies gained by treating health services as a standard unit of production will outweigh the fact that treating illness is a more variable and uncertain process than producing "widgets" in a factory.

The federal ESRD program was one of the first examples where the government allowed a private market to develop around the provision of publicly financed medical services. This chapter traces the history of these developments and the implications of the market influence on clinical decision making and patient experience.

The Market and Health

A proprietary model of illness and health care views disease in terms of its potential for economic growth. Health care, needed to "treat" the disease, becomes a commodity subject to the forces of the market. The patient becomes a consumer. The idea of health care as a commodity was praised by proponents as a "breakthrough"[1] in the health care industry, and at the same time was first condemned by critics as only furthering the interests of capital accumulation.[2] The implications of the commodification of health are particularly troubling in the chronic disease "market." First of all, business investments in health care are "technology-intensive" because highly technological solutions seem quite profitable to the firm. One of the reasons for this is the propensity toward monopolization in the health products industry. High-technology health care requires large capital investments, highly sophisticated facilities, and technically trained personnel. It is difficult for small firms to survive in such a market. The effect of monopolization in the high-technology health sector is, of course, price manipulation.

In its particular application to chronic illness, the market requires high disease incidence; increases in disease incidence spell economic expansion. Prevention is rarely considered, for such a concept would undercut the growth potential of the medical device and service industries. Related to this is another characteristic of the market model applied to health: social costs are externalized. Social costs, generally speaking, are the quality-of-life "costs" experienced by persons dependent on technological innovations for extended life. Such intangible costs, by no means insignificant, are considered "externalities" in economic terms and are rarely considered in corporate strategic planning for economic growth.

Federal Policy and the Market Conception of Health

Federal policy plays a key role in the market construction of health. Federal funding that subsidizes the privately run health care sector provides a base for economic growth. As such, investments in the health care industry can seem relatively safe, and stock ratings reflect this security. A predictable flow of federal funds gives confidence to investors, and the conventional rhetoric assures us that federal funding will further spur production, increase corporate taxes, and create jobs. Costs will be controlled if the market mechanisms of competition are allowed to operate. Rarely does this idealized version of market forces receive close enough scrutiny to test the validity of its assumption.

The financial cost of ESRD treatment was borne by the individual and/or the insurance company until 1972. Federal funding for ESRD treatment under the Medicare amendments ensured that everyone who needed treatment for kidney failure would have it. In this chapter, I will present profiles of the historical development (since 1972) of two private firms that operate in the dialysis industry or, as a prominent business magazine first put it, the "artificial kidney business."[3] These two firms represent the two sides of this business— the production of equipment necessary for dialysis, and the provision of dialysis itself in proprietary dialysis clinics. How do the principles of the market actually operate within this sector, and what effect has federal funding had on the development and growth of this industry? How does competition operate in these two sectors of the kidney business and at what cost to the kidney patient and the federal government?

The Medical Device Industry—Dialysis Equipment

The renal dialysis equipment industry is composed of those firms that manufacture and distribute equipment and supplies to hospitals, free-standing facilities, and home patients. The equipment and supplies include three kinds: (1) delivery and monitoring equipment, (2) dialyzers (or artificial kidneys), and (3) dialysis fluid, needles and syringes, blood tubing, and other miscellaneous disposable supplies.

The kidney machine is the hardware of hemodialysis. A complete dialysate delivery unit that includes the most advanced monitoring and control features   costed $5,000 to $6,000 in 1974. It is an expensive machine and represents a significant outlay of capital. Still, this product group is probably the smallest in terms of gross revenues among the hemodialysis-related product groups. In rough orders of magnitude, by 1975 there were more than 4,000 new patient stations manufactured and sold per annum, for gross industry revenues of approximately $20 to $25 million.[4]

The key to hemodialysis treatment, of course, is the artificial kidney. The sales of artificial kidneys, or dialyzers, alone represent almost one-half of all revenues from hemodialysis-related products. Indeed, dialyzers, along with other disposable equipment such as blood tubing, connectors, and needles, represent approximately 70 percent of the cost of hemodialysis treatment. These products accounted for nearly $200 million in sales or gross revenues per year after just three years of federal funding.[5]

There are several consumable supplies such as saline, heparin, and the dialysis fluid that, although relatively inexpensive per unit per treatment, actually added up to industry sales in excess of $50 million per annum by 1976.

Thus, we are describing an industry that, within five years of the establishment of federal reimbursements, generated yearly sales close to $300 million. Little is known, however, about the concentration ratio or the competitiveness of this industry. Perhaps regional or local markets might be characterized as monopolistic, which would have long-term implications for ESRD program costs.

Available data suggest that the industry was very concentrated almost from the start. Each of the major product groups was characterized by significant concentration of sellers. But because this is a relatively new industry, it is conceivable that initial observations were in a disequilibrium. However, early concentration of this industry represents a trend. In all three areas of equipment, major market concentration continues to the current time.

One important facet of the early stages of the dialysis industry and its products is that all three major product components were interrelated; dialysis equipment, however, usually could not be interchanged among different manufacturers. Changes during 1978 in FDA regulations made this restriction illegal, and new systems are now compatible with other manufacturers' supplies. Despite this regulation, however, doctors providing patient care have always tended to select and use equipment as much as possible from one or two suppliers for reasons of compatibility. Physicians have the primary decision-making responsibility for selection of renal dialysis equipment. The medical technicians who provide the day-to-day equipment maintenance are also heavily consulted about the purchase of delivery and monitoring equipment. One-time purchase products do not comprise the major portion of dollar sales. The primary purchase decision is the type of dialyzer that is to be used, for this decision influences all subsequent purchasing decisions.

The product differentiation within the industry is based more on reputation and reliability than on actual "consumer" experience. This is because a physician is reluctant to experiment with different types of equipment because of the possible life-or-death consequences of such an approach. Further, the ability of the supplier to provide a total package of equipment and service is an important decision factor.

We have some idea of the relative market shares of companies that provide kidney machines. Table 12 shows the sales and market shares for 1976.

This was clearly not a highly competitive industry, and appeared to be an oligopolistic industry, with the two largest firms having better than 50 percent of the market and the three largest sharing some 72.1 percent of the market among them. There has been little significant change in either the relative rankings of the apparent concentration ratio in recent years.

A somewhat similar pattern prevailed for the industry sales as a whole through 1976. Although a single company, Baxter Travenol, had twice the market share of the second largest firm in terms of gross sales, the four largest firms accounted for only 58.5 percent of all sales, as compared with an 81.4 percent of the market share for the

Table 12
The Market Performance of Manufacturers of
Hemodialysis Machines, 1976

Company	Sales Volume (thousands of $)	Market Share (%)
Drake Willock	6,500	30.2
Baxter Travenol	4,800	22.3
Cobe Laboratories	4,215	19.6
Extracorporeal	2,000	9.3
All others	3,985	18.6
Total	21,500	100.0

Source: Frost and Sullivan, *Analysis of the Market for Dialysis Equipment and Supplies* (New York: n. pub., 1977).

largest four in the case of kidney machines. Table 13 shows the competitive ranking of suppliers of hemodialysis-related products in the United States in 1976. As seen before, the figures do not describe a competitive industry. It is difficult, however, to find reliable sources of data to analyze competitive behaviors because renal product sales are often aggregated with all other medical devices that the company produces.

Table 13
The Market Performance of Manufacturers of
Hemodialysis-Related Products, 1976

Company	Sales (thousands of $)	Market Share (%)
Baxter Travenol	50,080	25.3
Cordis Dow	26,410	13.5
Extracorporeal	23,000	11.6
Cobe Laboratories	16,000	8.1
Gambro	12,000	6.1
Drake Willock	7,500	3.8
All others	62,465	31.6
Total	197,455	100.0

Source: Frost and Sullivan, *Analysis of the Market for Dialysis Equipment and Supplies* (New York: n. pub., 1977).

Technical change came very slowly to the industry during the mid-1970s. This is due in large part to the lack of desire on the part of many physicians for innovation and change. Technical changes tended to fall in the product improvement category rather than major change category (e.g., more reliable blood tubing or lower percentage of leaking dialyzers). The lack of major innovation and change within the industry has made it difficult for new manufacturers to market their products. The physician is in a high-risk situation and has tended to stay with the more reliable and proven products. Therefore, barriers to entry exist in this industry. A logical source of this barrier, in the equipment and supplies product groups, is the extent to which a given kidney machine can only, at best, operate with its own disposable equipment and supplies. A related but less restrictive potential barrier would be the marketing policy and customer service characteristics of the major machine manufacturers. This involves detail men extensively, much as does, for example, marketing in the drug industry.

Baxter Travenol—The Growth of the Industry Leader

Baxter Travenol, Inc. (formerly Baxter Laboratories), quickly became the largest producer of artificial kidneys, cornering some 40 percent of the total market by the mid-1970s. In addition to the dialysis machine itself, of which there are three types, the dialysis treatment requires a liquid solution of electrolytes, called a dialysate, which is pumped alongside the patient's blood, as well as several additional pieces of medical paraphernalia. Baxter manufactures a full line of kidney dialysis products, including the pump, bath tank, blood sets, blood leak detector, infusion pump, dialysate, and all of the three types of dialyzers—capillary flow, parallel flow, and coil.

Headquartered in Deerfield, Illinois, Baxter Travenol had twenty-nine domestic and twenty-four foreign operations, including those in South America and in Israel, the Philippines, and South Africa, in 1976. Its products were manufactured in fourteen different countries and sold in ninety countries.

Baxter produces medical care products that are used in a variety of medical treatments, not just in dialysis. Medical care products compose 94 percent of Baxter's business and can be divided into three groups. *Parenteral solutions* and *blood containers* include intravenous products, of which Baxter is also the leading manufacturer, irrigating solutions, and equipment used in the collection, process-ing, storage, and transfusion of blood and blood components. *Disposable administration sets* include a variety of plastic tubing connectors used in infusing parenteral solutions, in collecting and transfusing blood and blood components, and in kidney dialysis and heart-lung oxygenation. *Medical specialties* include kidney machine products, blood treatment and cardiopulmonary products, diagnos-tic reagents, drugs and pharmaceutical enzymes, medical gloves, medical instruments, miscellaneous disposable devices, plasma volume expanders, and urological products. Medical specialties com-pose 45 percent of total sales. As with other medical device manufac-turers, Baxter chose to concentrate in the highly profitable chronic disease and critical care products area. The remainder of Baxter's business is in enzymes and specialty chemicals with nonmedical applications (in food, brewing, textile, leather, laundry, and dry cleaning industries) and precision scientific instruments.

Baxter's sales and earnings records were outstanding during the 1960s and 1970s. Standard and Poor's company profile cited an "impressive record of long-term earnings growth," and the *Wall Street Journal* recommended the corporation as a sound investment and proclaimed it "an institutional darling" that "has dazzled Wall Street with its earnings prowess."[6]

Sales from 1972 through 1976 increased by 18.7 percent annu-ally, and from a volume of $37,562,000 in 1971 to a 1976 total of $564,085,000, or a total fifteen-fold increase. The annual report from 1976 cited a gross profit for 1975 of $234,478,000, or a profit margin of 41.6 percent (18 percent is generally considered a good profit margin) for the nine-month period ending 30 September 1976; net income rose 34.6 percent, and common stock rose from $1.04 to $1.34 per share. This company's activities were so sound that an offering of $100 million of new 25-year, 4¾ percent convertible debentures were "snapped up" by investors.[7] The debentures were rated BAA by Moody's (considered very good) and triple-B by Stan-dard and Poor's (also considered very good).

The *Wall Street Journal* praised Baxter's strong performance, attributable to "ongoing market expansion and new kidney dialysis products."[8] Baxter Travenol attributed its 1975 sales increase of over 18 percent primarily to higher prices, mostly in domestic markets. The gross profit margin increased 20 percent from 1974 to 1975, as opposed to 30 percent in the previous year. Baxter's 10-K report (a yearly report on the activities of a company required by the federal government) commented, "During each of the last three years, costs have risen somewhat more rapidly than sales."[9] Inflationary factors, they said, coupled with higher manufacturing costs to implement advancing quality control and product technology, resulted in higher costs in 1974 and particularly in 1975. Price increases initiated in 1974 and fully realized in 1975, and, to a lesser extent, additional 1975 price increases, moderated the impact of the foregoing factors.

A "Heard on the Street" column from the *Wall Street Journal* of 19 December 1974 provided further analysis of this situation.[10] The article quotes Michael M. LeConey, analyst at Faulkner, Dawkins & Sullivan, who claims that a substantial portion of the profit increase reported by hospital supply companies can be attributed to gains in the value of inventories.

Hospital supply has been a fast-growing industry. It has experienced strong productivity gains, which has minimized the need for price increases. For this reason, Mr. LeConey says, it hasn't reacted rapidly enough to the mounting pressure cost increases have put on profit margins. This is reflected in a decline in reported gross profit margins for most of the companies in the past two years, he adds.[11]

The Travenol price increases provide "compensation" for the pressure of inflationary costs, company officials add.[12]

One reason for the high net profits is that Baxter enjoyed tax-exempt status for operations in Ireland and Puerto Rico that amounted to 22 percent of the total manufacturing production. The company's 10-K report stated, "During the past three years the Company's effective tax rate has been approximately 20%." (This is in comparison with the average effective corporate U.S. tax rate of 48 percent.) This tax rate is attributable principally to the benefit arising from the tax exemptions granted to the company by the governments of Puerto Rico and Ireland to encourage establishment of operations in those locations.[13] Baxter paid a total of $11,119,000 in income taxes for fiscal 1975; the figure represents a 20 percent tax rate on stated earnings, and less than 2 percent of net sales, or less than 5 percent of gross profit.

Baxter was not the only company to firm up its competitive position by capitalizing on Irish tax incentives for foreign investment. According to the *Wall Street Journal* of 31 March 1975, most major pharmaceutical and hospital equipment companies have located operations in Ireland. The Irish government offers a fifteen-year exemption from Irish taxes and makes grants available as well. Ireland has been especially attractive to medical industries for a number of reasons.

> The Irish development group says that drugs and similar products have a "high added-value content," which means that they can be produced from inexpensive Irish raw materials and turned, by high technology processes, into products that can be sold at a considerably higher price. What's more, there's little bulk involved, so transportation costs to the Continent aren't an important consideration, as they would be for high-bulk, low-technology products.
>
> There's also the availability of relatively low paid, yet highly skilled workers, including scientists and technicians from Irish universities. Other countries might offer lower wage scales, drug firm executives say, but they don't offer the amount of education and literacy found in Ireland.

The article went on to say that Ireland's exports of drugs and fine chemicals increased dramatically, from $4.5 million in 1965 to over $140 million a year in 1974, "up almost 300% in the past four years alone."[14] Baxter's annual report for 1975 acknowledged that the company

> had uncovered foreign questionable payments made principally to relatives of government employees. The payments occurred mainly in one country and were not material in terms of the company's worldwide operations. A Special Committee of the Board of Directors found that the senior management of the company had no prior knowledge of the payments and that there had been no illegal political contributions.[15]

An article appearing in the *Wall Street Journal*, however, claimed that payments of over $2.1 million were made to foreign countries over a five-year period. Citing a Baxter spokesman, the article stated that 97 percent of that money was spent in one country (unidentified). The largest contribution in any one year was $562,000, related to sales of $5.5 million, or a total payment of 10 percent of sales (reflecting a still substantial profit margin). According to the Baxter spokesman, $1,971,600 was "paid as commission-type payments in six countries, principally to relatives of government employees. Another $136,000 was paid in three countries to obtain payment of past due receivables for products sold to government agencies."[16]

Baxter Travenol gained near-monopoly control over the market in dialysis equipment through the use of its patents. Baxter holds patents for many of its products throughout the world, but, the company claims, it "does not consider any one or more of its patents . . . to be essential to its business."[17] Yet, in 1973, Baxter filed suit against Vernitron Corporation, another manufacturer of kidney dialysis products, for patent infringement when Vernitron tried to manufacture dialysis products that Baxter was also manufacturing. Vernitron, in turn, proposed to sue Baxter for antitrust violations. Baxter Travenol was forced to back down because its use of patents did, in fact, violate antitrust laws. In February 1976 the Vernitron Corporation announced that it had agreed in principle to settle the litigation.

> The proposal to settle all the litigation calls for a Vernitron subsidiary to be licensed under certain of Baxter's U.S. and foreign patents for artificial kidneys, or dialysis coils. A Baxter subsidiary would become a nonexclusive distributor of Vernitron's central-system kidney-dialysis equipment, which uses the coils. Vernitron said the distribution contract would guarantee, subject to certain financial penalties, that Baxter would sell a minimum of $4 million of Vernitron equipment over five years retroactive to January 1.[18]

The research and development funds of 1975—$26,839,000—represented an increase of 25 percent over 1974. Research and development expenditures maintained pace with sales increases at a level of between 4.6 percent and 5.2 percent of net sales from 1970 through 1975. The 10-K report for 1975 defined company research and development policy as follows:

> The Company follows a policy of concentrating on clearly defined areas of research and development, such as the collection, processing and preservation of blood, intravenous nutrition and therapy, kidney dialysis and cardiovascular diseases. Projects which are aimed at developing products for the market within two or three years are emphasized.[19]

Although it is not possible to get figures from the company on specific aspects of its product development, including the rate of obsolescence of old products, a sampling from fiscal year 1975 of new products for kidney dialysis and improvement on old products should give an idea of how the process of development works.

In 1975 Baxter Travenol introduced the Travenol CF Capillary Flow Dialyzer, which employs hollow fibers for exchange between blood and dialysate solution. The hollow-fiber method was first developed by a joint venture of the Cordis Corporation and Dow Chemical Company. Introduction of this type of dialyzer makes Baxter, in its chairman's words, "the only company to offer the physician all three basic methods for artificial kidney therapy."[20] Improvements were introduced in both parallel flow and coil dialyzers. According to a company brochure, "The new Travenol CD Coil Dialyzer has special new features designed to increase reliability, provide assured performance . . . and the new slim case makes it easier to handle and use."[21]

Product development in artificial kidneys for Baxter Travenol in one year consisted of duplicating a third model of dialysis machine, providing attractive and slim holding cases, introducing bath features that reduce splashing, and making remote control switches. All of these so-called product developments, one could argue, are fairly superficial and insignificant technological advances in dialysis treatment technology. These changes are, however, "growth stimulators" for Baxter Travenol.[22]

As the case of Baxter Travenol illustrates, dialysis equipment producers operated in a sector of the medical device industry where only the larger firms prospered because of demands for high volume and the money for research and development. A few fast-growing conglomerates bought out or merged with other companies.

Pricing Policies

An important characteristic of the industry is that price competition is rather limited. Competition tends to be across other dimensions of the products besides price. This is true in the equipment for delivery and monitoring of dialysis, which are capital expenditures that are amortized over a long period of time, and so cost alternatives are not frequently reviewed. In addition, the physician has the ability to demand a particular type of delivery or montoring system. For disposable supplies, the hospitals and home dialysis patients have concentrated on ease of ordering and convenience rather than on price. The government as primary payer tends to intensify this non-price competition. The fact that the federal reimbursement screen remained constant for ten years indicates that significant slack was built into the reimbursement structure from the start.

The research and development activities of these companies concentrated on the production of disposable products and a calculated rate of technological obsolescence.[23] Most analysts seemed to concur that the manufacture of dialysis equipment is a growth industry. Its prosperity was premised on a close link to federal dollars. The business press notes: "The key to future growth for this industry remains the funding sources."[24] In a private report one industry analyst says, "For those supplying the kidney machine . . . the potential is vast."[25]

Proprietary Clinics

The vast majority of ESRD patients were treated in a voluntary hospital setting during the early years of the federal program. However, private proprietary dialysis clinics in 1985 treated nearly 40 percent of ESRD patients. How can the growth of this business be examined? There are a number of private proprietary satellite clinics, but the largest has always been National Medical Care (NMC). As of 1978, NMC already administered nearly 1 million dialysis treatments and served nearly 20 percent of all ESRD patients in the country. In 1983, NMC operated 164 centers, with revenues increasing from $9 million in 1974 to 311 million in 1983.

NMC started as a conglomerate operating many different medical care ventures. In addition to operating satellite dialysis centers, NMC also operated in-patient mental health centers, out-patient mental health centers, residential treatment centers for retarded children, and skilled nursing facilities. However, the dialysis business quickly became the major source of revenues for NMC enterprises.

NMC began under a strong philosophy of the "efficiency-enhancing" ability of private enterprise. Its founders, chairman Constantine L. Hampers, M.D., and president Eugene Schupak, M.D., considered NMC to be "the first organization to provide a major breakthrough in health care delivery."[26] The breakthrough they described was the application of vigorous business techniques to the field of health care. Both founders were kidney specialists trained in the Regional Medical Program at Harvard who said that they went into private enterprise because they were dissatisfied with the non-profit hospital setting, particularly with its inability to provide cost-effective care. "Elements of solving the problems of treating E.S.R.D. have been at hand for years. Yet missing was a sound, economically feasible model for developing a health care system capable of keeping pace with rapidly changing elements within each of these disciplines."[27]

Schupak started his first private dialysis unit in Long Island City, Queens, in 1970. NMC grew dramatically since that year, largely because of the funding provided for hemodialysis by the Social Security Amendments of 1972. Dr. Schupak received quite a bit of bad press for his entrepreneurial zeal. A *New York Times* article in 1975 reported his attempt to corner the New York dialysis market with the help of an influential state senator.[28] What he sought was an exclusive contract with the city that would guarantee him all of the dialysis patients, except those who were acutely ill and whose care would then be costly. For-profit dialysis clinics contract with private as well as municipal hospitals to provide dialysis treatment for their ESRD patients. Schupak claimed he could save New York City $797,910 a year. A subsequent New York City Health Department study concluded that this arrangement would actually cost the city $103,280 a year. In response, Dr. Schupak claimed that the city hospitals were "turf conscious."[29]

By 1976 NMC's annual report to stockholders could make this claim:

> National Medical Care is the largest and most efficient single provider of artificial kidney services in the country. We have managed to maintain a reasonable profit despite escalating costs of supplies and personnel through the application of sensible, carefully controlled business procedures. We have achieved this through techniques such as standardization of supplies, volume buying, better personnel utilization, etc., procedures well-known to industry but heretofore rarely used in health care. Without depersonalization, we have been able to industrialize one segment of health care while improving patient care, but never accepting as dogma those procedures or techniques which could not be logically defended.[30]

The company's early growth record allowed little room for arguing against the financial soundness of this enterprise for investors.

The financial picture over the first five years after 1971 was dramatic. The five-year summary of operations shows an increase in general revenues from $9,400,218 in 1971 to $77,875,572 in 1975. Most of this growth is attributed to increases in the number of dialysis treatments given per year: 30,000 in 1971 to nearly 400,000 in 1976.[31]

The growth of the sales and manufacturing division of NMC, Erika, was equally dramatic. Sales outside the NMC operations climbed from less than $1 million in 1971 to more than $17 million in 1975, with an increase of 77 percent, or $7,431,000, from 1974 to 1975. Growth in Erika sales in 1975 also reflected an expansion into international markets. Offices were opened in Brussels and Toronto, NMC's first overseas ventures.

In sum, NMC's operations grew considerably, particularly after the advent of federal funding for dialysis. A closer look at the corporation's activities indicated that dialysis treatment was the most potentially lucrative, and NMC tried to integrate the whole operation vertically.

An interesting example of vertical integration was the manufacturing division of NMC, Erika. Erika is an integral part of NMC's operations. NMC wholly owns Erika, which is a major distributor of artificial kidney supplies and also manufactures an artificial kidney. Erika solved a perceived logistical problem of a catastrophic supply cut-off, according to the company:

> It is vital for National Medical Care to assure itself of a continued flow of all supplies and materials necessary for safe effective dialysis, in spite of such commonly encountered industrial problems such as work stoppages, production delays, and unsatisfactory manufacturing, in addition to power failure, water main breaks, and other such problems.[32]

Erika was portrayed as the solution to these potential problems. However, such catastrophes have never been encountered in other dialysis facilities that do not have manufacturing capabilities. This vertical integration seems to have had more to do with profit structure than with possible shortages. The divestitures of NMC during the mid-1970s, along with its growing capability to manufacture dialysis equipment, suggested that NMC attempted to create a vertical monopoly of dialysis treatment.

Further evidence of this trend toward monopolization was the fact that NMC was also involved in home dialysis, through Erika's operations. Through Erika, NMC distributes hemodialysis equipment to home dialysis patients and is currently the largest distributor of these products. Sales to home patients are initiated through institutional users, such as hospitals, and are made by prescription only. Erika's salesmen work directly with the home patient once the initial sale has been made. Erika had a sales catalogue prepared especially for home patient use and a home-dialysis kit that provides for an all-inclusive single shipment once every two months.

According to the company's 1976 10-K report, Erika competed for home dialysis sales principally with Travenol and Cope Laboratories. More than half of Erika's dialysis products were purchased from Travenol, and "Erika believes that it is the largest single customer for Travenol's dialysis products."[33] Sales were made under a "nonexclusive Distribution Agreement from 1972": "Either party may terminate the Distribution Agreement on 60 days' prior written notice, provided, however, if the agreement is so terminated by Travenol, it must pay Erika, for a period of 12 months following such termination, 10% of Travenol's net sales to certain accounts developed by Erika."[34]

NMC's satellite dialysis centers are also involved with home dialysis care. All of the centers "have home dialysis training teams and active training and support programs for home dialysis when medically indicated."[35] Although NMC had gotten into the home dialysis business, it did not believe (at this time) that home dialysis should be the predominant mode of treatment for ESRD patients. The company's executives supported an expansion in satellite-center treatment. As one annual report put it:

Home dialysis . . . has traditionally been described as being far less expensive than in-center or out-of-hospital satellite dialysis and adaptable to practically every home. Unfortunately, although it offers a distinct advantage in some cases, it cannot be applied to all patients and costs much more than people think.[36]

The report estimates that only 10 percent to 35 percent of patients are suitable for home dialysis and goes on to describe home dialysis as a "middle-class procedure" that is difficult for inner-city dwellers because of the physical facilities and the burden on family.[37] A rather poor analogy is drawn between home dialysis and home childbirth in an effort to demonstrate that home dialysis is not for everyone. The report also cited "a demonstrable increase in complications among home dialysis patients" and claims that the cost of home dialysis would be substantially increased if hospital costs for treatment complications (which run as high as 15 percent in some areas) were included. "When we add the cost of dialyzing these patients in the hospital (the most expensive form of dialysis) the true annualized cost of home dialysis comes very close to the cost of limited care center dialysis."[38] Of course, this same percentage of complications may arise for in-center, limited-care facilities, such as those operated by NMC. Many dialysis patients of either treatment modality require in-patient care from time to time because of dietary indiscretions and acute illness.

Many of the problems with home dialysis identified by NMC are in fact real. But it is also the case that limited-care facilities such as the satellite clinics are very profitable for the corporation. It is therefore difficult to separate out the motivations of the corporate executives with respect to home dialysis. The expansion of satellite dialysis centers has been subject to heavy criticism. In part, this is because it represents the most blatantly profit-making aspect of ESRD care, in a field where the government is the largest source of direct finance. A second reason is in the trend of satellite centers to take away from the hospitals the least complicated (and hence most profitable) ESRD cases, leaving hospitals with the complex, acute, and expensive ones. NMC itself as much as stated this when giving a prognostication of business trends:

> National Medical Care expected limited care dialysis to continue to expand rapidly and anticipated that hospital dialysis will remain about the same in total volume, but will show a *large increase* in acute, or "back-up" dialysis, and a major *decrease in dialysis of chronic, stable* out-patients.[39]

National Medical Care saw little possibility of a decrease in the incidence of ESRD and consider prospects for prevention as "dim." It was also lukewarm toward transplants and predicted that transplantation would not show much of an improved batting average.[40] Generally, NMC has always predicted that the number of persons requiring dialysis will continue to increase. Rising incidence of renal disease, then, is linked to corporate viability for NMC.

NMC has displayed an interesting ambiguity toward federal involvement in ESRD. Although it considered organized federal funding to be a "major breakthrough," it warned that "obstacles can be introduced by well-intentioned but unrealistic government regulations."[41] Yet government and industry are very closely allied in ESRD treatment. A former vice-president in charge of research and governmental relations for NMC was Dr. Charles Edwards. An example of the "revolving door" tendency of executives to move back and forth from government to industry, Dr. Edwards was the former assistant secretary for health of DHEW. It was during Dr. Edward's tenure in government that the amendments to Medicare in 1972 that established federal funding for ESRD treatment were passed and the reimbursement regulations, so favorable for NMC's growth, were established.

It is impossible to separate the growth of this industry from the logic of federal intervention. Both appear to be only different facets of common assumptions concerning medical care and the private market. The federal health logic that generally promotes technological solutions to complex social problems is inherently biased toward resource-intensive approaches that pump funds into the industrial sector. At the same time, this logic of health policy disparages the excessive costs of a high-tech-oriented health care system. This is a conscious but enduring contradiction of federal health policy.

The Dialysis Business since 1978: Servicing the $1.8 Billion Market

The market in ESRD equipment and supplies has changed in some important ways during the last six years, but many of the trends established during the early 1970s still hold. The larger companies that could divide the market among themselves have had to contend with aggressive new entries. Some of the old firms have been forced to drop out of the race for an increasing market share. In fact, there has been a demise of the small independent dialysis firms and an increase in the large and diversified pharmaceutical firms. Such corporate giants as Johnson & Johnson and Eli Lilly have entered the market, mostly through acquisitions of existing smaller firms. Because the growth rate of the ESRD population has slowed down during the last few years, the marketing efforts of the major companies have intensified. They can no longer rely on a rapidly increasing number of patients to fuel corporate growth.

A particularly important change has been the integration of equipment and disposable supplies as a manufacturing strategy for a company. Further, individual companies are producing both hemodialysis and peritoneal dialysis products, a departure from the earlier period when separate companies specialized in one or the other product line.[42] Thus, a strategy of intense marketing of a full line of products characterizes the larger firms. A company can use a strong product as the "hook" to sell other products that might not be as attractive.

Baxter Travenol continues to be the leader in this field, as indicated in Table 14. Baxter controls 38 percent of the disposable market and 34 percent of the equipment market. Though a host of younger companies are providing aggressive competition, Baxter is well positioned to continue as an industry leader and strongly influences the shape of the supply business. The company is large, well capitalized, competes in international markets, and has the manufacturing capacity to produce new product lines when a new market develops. With 1982 sales of $1.7 billion and sales increases of 40 percent a year since 1978, Baxter's stock price has climbed dramatically. During 1983 the price went from $34.75 a share to $60 a share. Baxter increasingly looks to the international market for future growth possibilities. (Joint ventures are under discussion with both the Yugoslavian and Chinese governments.)

CAPD: The Low-Cost Solution to the Federal Government's Problems?

During this period of federal concern with "unanticipated costs," a number of firms have begun to promote CAPD (continuous ambulatory peritoneal dialysis) as the optimum approach. During the late 1970s Baxter, Abbot, and later Delmed developed CAPD product lines with Baxter—until recently, the only producer of the sterile solution used in this procedure. These firms lobbied Congress and HCFA very aggressively, convincing the government of the cost effectiveness of CAPD. This assumption of a new technological cost-fix was a major consideration when the government decided to drop the reimbursement rates for ESRD treatment in 1983. HCFA even included a passage in these regulations that says: "CAPD is the preferred method of treatment for many patients."[43] Support for such a judgment was based on highly contestable data. No controlled clinical trial comparing CAPD with hemodialysis exists. Most information on the effectiveness of CAPD comes either from physicians

Table 14

Competitive Standings in the Hemodialysis Markets, 1981

Company	Disposables ($)*	% of Total	Equipment ($)†	% of Total	Total ($)	% of Total
Baxter Travenol	78,500	38.0	2,500	8.0	81,000	34.0
B-D Drake Willock	—	—	9,400	30.0	9,400	4.0
Cobe Laboratories	27,500	13.3	14,200	45.0	41,700	17.5
Cordis Dow	40,000	19.3	—	—	40,000	16.7
Extracorporeal Medical Specialties	26,900	13.0	1,600	5.0	28,500	12.0
Gambro	20,700	10.0	—	—	20,700	8.7
Other	13,200	6.4	3,800	12.0	17,000	7.1

*Disposables include dialyzers, tubing, connectors, and needles.
†Equipment includes water purification systems.
Source: Frost and Sullivan, *Analysis of the Market for Dialysis Equipment and Supplies* (New York: n. pub., 1981).

who promote the modality or from the companies that produce the CAPD equipment.

The quality-of-care and safety issues that are so important in the assessment of a new technology are clearly secondary to the cost-control imperatives. One HCFA staffer made this clear: "If patients want that treatment because it frees them from a machine, and if doctors are going to prescribe it, then as long as it costs less we'll endorse it. It's not up to us to judge the technology."[44] The best evidence available indicates that the rate of complications for CAPD is 50 percent higher than for hemodialysis, but the siren's song of lower costs will always lead the federal government into dangerous waters. It is a lesson in how quickly low-cost products directly influence the dynamics of patient care. This new procedure is used increasingly in ESRD facilities all over the country, increasing at a rate of 20 percent a year.[45] In 1983, 12 percent of all dialysis patients used this modality. This is because government reimbursement rates force facilities to use the cheapest modalities available to hold costs down. Many ESRD nurses feel that the patient bears the experiential costs of these policies in increased morbidity and mortality.

Such policies are technology-forcing in a negative sense. As I indicated in Chapter 1, even clinical considerations, let alone social ones, begin to play a secondary role when the market dominates the policy discourse. It becomes difficult to get an objective assessment of so-called cost-effective technologies such as CAPD. The rhetoric of cost containment provides a momentum and an ideological dominance of criticism of the risks involved. A concern for quality of care is rapidly becoming a label for soft thinking about the "tough" problems of efficient program management. "Without cost control there might be no program" is the unspoken, but all too clear, message of the current federal administration. A return to the "death committees" is the specter that lurks in the background, another version of the death-or-life dichotomy that so powerfully shapes policies in health. This is doubly unfortunate. For one thing, current federal policies, strongly influenced by the myth of the market, do in fact impose the tragic choices of the death committees. The only difference is that the government claims to offer care in a democratic and equitable manner based on need when, in reality, it places through market mechanisms a selective pressure on those patients with extreme needs and costly care. It does this by simply restricting the resources available to facilities that treat complex patients, generally the hospitals. The market is an effective and mostly silent triage device; tragic choices are not clearly visible as public problems. The second issue is ironic; these market initiatives rarely control costs at all, even with the quality "tradeoffs" that the program managers are willing to accept. Firms in the kidney business are built on government revenues and, more often than not, bite the hand that feeds them, or at least try. A case in point is the most recent success story of the kidney business, Delmed, whose chairman Amin Khoury stated, "Profit used to be a bad thing in medicine. Now it isn't."[46]

Delmed certainly knows something about fast profits. This company, founded in 1974, went public in 1981. Annual sales have doubled during the last three years, from $30 million to more than $60 million, on the strength of its peritoneal dialysis products.[47] Delmed is currently second only to Baxter Travenol in the "hot" peritoneal market, one that is expected to grow to more than $600 million in sales by 1986. Baxter now refuses to sell supplies to Delmed; why support the competition? This has forced Delmed to use a foreign supplier of dialysate solution, raising some problems for the company later. *Barron's*, the business weekly published by Dow Jones Company, published an article on the questionable practices (both business and ethical) of Delmed. On the ethical side, the article stated that the company offered "rebates" (kickbacks) to the dialysis facilities that have their patients buy supplies directly from Delmed rather than through the hospital. This practice allowed Delmed to charge a dialysis patient a price that was three times the hospital charge. Delmed then returned a portion of this profit to the ESRD facility as a "rebate."[48] HCFA sent out a notice to all facilities specifying that such acts might be "in violation of a criminal statute."[49] The *Barron's* article further stated that Delmed's foreign plant was not licensed by the FDA to produce dialysis solution for sale in this country because it failed to meet standards of good manufacturing practices.[50]

In the rush to get a jump on this government-dependent market in peritoneal dialysis, Delmed took on heavy corporate debts. These have been reported to be as large as seven times their equity level (the company owes seven times the value of its cashable assets). Following his own advice on profits in medicine mentioned earlier, Delmed's chief executive officer Khoury sold personal holdings of nearly $800,000 in Delmed stocks during 1983 and 1984.

The Profit-making Dialysis Business

In 1985, National Medical Care continued to dominate the market for proprietary dialysis. Revenues increased from $190 million in 1979 to $311 million in 1983. The industry trend toward CAPD and the changes in federal reimbursement policies for ESRD in 1983 (the reimbursement issues will be discussed in more detail in Chapter 7) worked together to emphasize home dialysis over center-based services. These changes suggested that NMC would face the prospect of diminishing earnings under the current regulatory environment.

In the annual report of 1983 the officers of NMC presented a new marketing strategy that they hoped would be effective in the competitive environment that they labeled a "revolution in health care."[51] Dr. C. L. Hampers, chairman, president, and chief executive officer of the company, described NMC's opposition to the regulatory changes that he considered "contrary to the interests of effective medical care."[52] Because of these changes the company experienced an average net realizable rate per treatment that was $6.70 lower than previous levels for their in-patient services. The rate that the government paid for home dialysis, however, was higher than before. In a reversal of the corporate rhetoric that had characterized their annual reports for over a decade, NMC now fully embraced home dialysis and increased their rate of home dialysis treatments.

A most interesting part of NMC's marketing efforts was their attempt to reach out to nonprofit hospitals and other dialysis providers. Dr. Hampers stated:

> We recognize that the greatest burden of change has fallen upon the many hospitals and other providers of dialysis who are being reimbursed below their costs. . . . The company has an unique opportunity to expand its dialysis service . . . to meet the needs of other providers. To that end our dialysis services division has mounted an ambitious marketing effort to offer our dialysis services to hospitals which can benefit from our expertise.[53]

The goal, then, was to capture some of the hospital-based dialysis market.

NMC has diversified into eight wholly owned subsidiaries, including its dialysis services division (Bio-medical Applications, or BMA), dialysis products (Erika and LifeChem, which performs blood testing for patients), Gluco-Med (out-patient diabetes centers), Dartmouth

Insurance Company, MedTech (respiratory and rehabilitation therapy products), and Theranutrix (infusion therapies to home patients including nutritional support and chemotherapy). In August of 1984 NMC became part of W. R. Grace and Co., a multi-billion-dollar corporation that was originally an international leader in speciality chemicals. As part of Grace's diversification strategy, they joined such companies as Herman's World of Sporting Goods, El Torito Restaurants, and Channel Home Centers. Grace bought 49 percent of NMC and the management took the rest in a leveraged buy-out arrangement.

Why did Grace enter the advanced medical products field? The company's executive vice-president Terrence D. Daniels commented, "Dialysis separates out the impurities in the blood of a kidney patient. . . . The technology is now being developed to do this with other diseases."[54] The company thinks that dialysis techniques can be used in the treatment of multiple sclerosis although such applications are controversial. Grace also owns Amicon Corp., a manufacturer of synthetic membranes that is at work on an artificial pancreas. The company in November purchased 5 percent of Symbion, Inc., the firm established by Dr. Robert Jarvik and the maker of the artificial heart. Grace obviously sees the artificial organ market as a lucrative business.

The merger of NMC with a large corporate monolith increases the pressures on the company to stress short-run profitability. The effect of this on their dialysis services should be an important concern to federal officials who manage the ESRD program.

Questionable Assumptions of State Policy

It is evident that a number of the assumptions of health policy with respect to the provision of ESRD services must be reexamined. First of all, the assumption that costs will be controlled by competition in the market is clearly wrong. Firms in the artificial kidney business tend toward monopolization, both vertically and horizontally. As discussed in the chapter on the legislative history, recent federal concerns regarding the ESRD program under Medicare center primarily on rising costs, which is totally predictable from the foregoing analysis. Yet policy makers have no explanation other than inflation or inefficiency for the "run-away costs" of dialysis treatment.

A second assumption of state policy that calls for the public subsidy of the health care industry is that subsidization is a spur to economic growth and will be returned to the economy in the form of jobs and corporate income taxes. Yet, as is evident at least in the case of Baxter-Travenol, industry avoids taxes by relocating its manufacturing activity to foreign countries. With these relocations go the jobs.

These findings suggest that medical care interventions can often be influenced by the industrial policies of private firms. The government considers this either as benign or, during the Reagan administration, as a positive force of rational efficiency. Federal policy is similar in other Medicaid programs, such as nursing homes, or home health, where the private market increasingly dominates the provision of care. Policy continues in this direction, in the face of continual evidence of the inadequacy of this model. In the following chapter I will look closely at the realities of the market in the provision of ESRD services. Do we see a rational and cost-effective approach to catastrophic health care needs consistent with the public's interest? Or, in fact, does the myth of market rationality represent an ideal, but unrealized vision?

CHAPTER SEVEN

Corporate Influence and the Politics of Research

On 10 May 1983 I received a letter from the senior vice-president of National Medical Care, E. G. Lowrie, M.D. It arrived in dramatic fashion: special delivery certified mail requiring a return receipt. The letter stated (in part):

I am deeply concerned about your analytic method and submit that it presents a highly distorted image of the facts. My reasons for so stating are outlined below. But I am doubly concerned because HCFA (who funded your study) has been trying unsuccessfully for some time to allege skewed case mix between hospital and for-profit, non-hospital units. Insomuch as your analysis allegedly supports that thesis, they might reasonably be expected to both support and use it.

National Medical Care owns and operates three of the five for-profit, non-hospital units in Michigan. Reporting data to HCFA which has been distorted by statistical analysis and publishing it in a journal with high press visibility such as the *New England Journal of Medicine* will do National Medical Care irreparable harm. I have therefore been advised by counsel to review my discussion with you in writing. In addition to our talk, I have reviewed two typescripts listing you as first author. The first of these is a technical description titled, "Initial Patient Characteristics and Risk in End Stage Renal Disease: The Development of Severity Groupings through Survival Analysis". The second is clearly intended for publication and discusses case mix differences between hospitals and independents.

This is not an issue involving freedom of the press or public expression of opinion. The Brandeis Health Policy Consortium and you will be regarded as expert and you have sufficient technical expertise to evaluate these data objectively and to report their results in an unbiased and direct way. Please be advised that we intend to submit your study for detailed statistical consultation, evaluation, and review and will seek the appropriate remedies if our perceptions are confirmed.

Why was this multimillion dollar corporation so concerned with the implications of this ongoing research? What prompted the thinly veiled threat of legal action? How had Dr. Lowrie acquired early drafts of a paper I was preparing to submit for publication?

This chapter considers the political economy of health care research. The rise of profit-making firms in the health care system makes it very likely that health policy research findings will have implications for some corporation's bottom line. Firms like NMC are almost totally dependent on federal reimbursement for operating revenues. Research findings that suggest changes in levels of payment for ESRD are of more than passing interest to them. How does a corporation attempt to influence the research that is the basis for policy decisions?

In the characteristically myopic framework of federal policy, the question "who is treating whom and at what costs?" has dominated the discussion of ESRD since 1980. Increasingly, this federal program is cited as an example of runaway costs. A program initially based (at least rhetorically) on human compassion has changed to one in which efficiency and cost effectiveness reign as the principal organizing logics. As I indicated in Chapter 6, the ideal of a competitive market for ESRD services, initially championed by the corporations that make up the "dialysis business," has become de facto federal policy.

Much of the debate surrounding these issues takes place in the mass media and professional journals. It is very much a "public policy issue," but the shaping of the problems and the nature of debate is influenced by the dialectic of the market and the clinic. Considerations of actual human experience with the technology are either ignored or oversimplified. The public issues cannot embrace the complexity and texture of the private experience of ESRD. The story is diffused across the terrain of medical research journals, policy analysis, congressional hearings, and financial reporting.

I want to draw together the various "angles" of this story in this chapter, to reconstruct the cultural whole from the social fragments that typify a "policy problem." From this a pattern will emerge, elucidating connections between the apparently separate problems of market, science, politics, and experience.

Reimbursement and Cost Containment: The Application of Market Fixes

The cost of the ESRD program has risen at a much faster rate than was predicted. In 1972 Congress was told that the program would cost $250 million per year at the end of four years.[1] Instead, the cost was twice that, and by 1983 expenditures had soared to approximately $1.7 billion.

Escalating costs have become almost the single focus of the Reagan administration's health policy, and problems within the ESRD program have been reduced to fit this frame. There has been a hectic search to find the culprit behind the treatment program's high costs. The increase is usually attributed to many different "culprits": (1) the high rates Medicare pays for dialysis in ESRD facilities; (2) a lack of incentives to encourage Medicare patients to choose less expensive methods of treatment such as kidney transplants and home dialysis; (3) significant growth in the ESRD populations; and (4) the repetitive nature of the treatment for a chronic condition.[2]

Many of HCFA's efforts at containing costs have encouraged the use of what are believed to be less costly treatments (home dialysis, CAPD, and transplantation). There is limited and contradictory evidence about the cost of any one mode of treatment, and controversy as to which modes cost less continues.[3] It has also been difficult to develop purely economic incentives for the use of these modes. The clinical decision as to whether a patient is suitable for transplantation, for example, resides ideally with patients and their physicians and surgeons. It is not the province for government policy, but there have been continual efforts to increase federal legislative involvement in patient care decisions in the name of cost control. In 1977 legislative efforts to remove disincentives to home dialysis were thwarted by a strong lobby representing the proprietary dialysis industry (the lobbying was partially financed by NMC). During that year the House Ways and Means Committee tried to cut costs by proposing a bill that would have required almost half of all dialysis patients to be treated at home. NMC hired John Sears, former Reagan campaign manager, as a lobbyist. Through his efforts, the proposal was essentially gutted; its language was reduced to a simple acknowledgment of the suitability of home dialysis in limited cases: "the maximum practical number of patients who are medically, socially, and psychologically suitable candidates for home dialysis or transplantation should be so treated."[4]

John Sears's pitch was, "What's wrong with making a profit?"[5] The interesting contradiction is that the rationale of cost containment and efficiency espoused by HCFA was at odds with the internal logic of private capital. NMC, a firm that makes its business treating patients in large private facilities, stood to lose money if large numbers of patients were switched to home treatment, no matter how efficient this might be from the government's perspective. Through a neat twist of logic, NMC publicly argued that the government would violate the doctor-patient relationship by mandating the use of a particular mode of treatment. Further, NMC considered that forcing patients to be treated by a specific technology violated their rights and could adversely affect the quality of care.

NMC learned from this episode that the rhetoric of clinical concern was persuasive in protecting their corporate interests. It also seemed apparent that the federal government suspected that NMC's rapid growth was related to overgenerous payment rates. Obviously, the corporation needed to provide hard data to dispel such suspicions and "prove" that profit-making dialysis was efficient or even superior to other alternatives. This would involve a strategy of establishing a "scientific" basis for the cost effectiveness of for-profit care.

As the controversy of cost-effective dialysis moved into public debate, the strategy of proving the "efficiency" of a particular technology more by effective public relations than by empirically validated research would evolve. A two-part article appeared in *Science*, setting the tone for the ideological battle. *Science* writer Gina Kolata investigated the profits of NMC and found that "NMC thrives selling dialysis."[6] This was one of the first articles to raise the issue of the growing profit-making sector that was not written in the business press for potential investors. Kolata's article was followed closely by an article in the *New England Journal of Medicine* entitled "The New Medical-Industrial Complex."[7] Written by Arnold S. Relman, the journal's editor, it called attention to an "un-precedented phenomenon with broad and troubling implications for the future of our medical care system."[8] He highlighted NMC as an example of the way that private enterprise was stimulated by public funding of health care, raising the question of "cream skimming" by proprietary facilities.

My initial recommendation, therefore, is that we should pay more attention to the new health-care industry. It needs to be studied carefully, and its performance should be measured and compared with that of the nonprofit sector. We need to know much more about the quality and cost of the services provided by the profit-making companies on use, distribution, and access. We also must find out the extent to which "cream-skimming" is occurring and whether competition from profit-making providers is really threatening the survival of our teaching centers and major urban hospitals.[9]

This same issue of the journal carried another article, this one specifically about the ESRD program. "Treatment of End-Stage Renal Disease: Free but Not Equal" by Relman and Rennie used federal data indicating that the rate of dialysis in the United States was much higher than in Europe.[10] Their main concern was to consider the role of profit-making dialysis in our increasing use of this technology. Might the profit motive account for this expanding use of dialysis? There are "suggestions that commercialism may have a role," concluded the authors, but more data is required to make a clear judgment.[11]

Thus the challenge was raised and the battle begun over the role of the profit-making sector in the medical care system in general and in ESRD in particular. The battles would be waged on the pages of research journals and articulated through the mass media. The rhetorical lines were drawn: clinical versus corporate control of medical technology. Although the debate would be framed in terms of the patient's "needs" or in the name of equitable policies, it represented a classic contest between a traditional professional elite (academic doctors) and the brash advocates of private market efficiency. The federal government's policies were passively dependent on the outcome.

Data, Data, Who's Got the Data?

Obtaining accurate data about the cost of the ESRD program has been and continues to be extremely difficult. Although all ESRD facilities are required to submit cost reports to HCFA, compliance is not perfect and variations in reported cost allocations make it difficult to perform comparative analyses. A recent audit of 110 facilities showed up to a 15 percent difference between reported and actual facility costs.[12] In 1972, when the federal program began, there was little information on which to base fair rates of reimbursement. There were large differences in charges for dialysis and transplantation services in different facilities, and these did not necessarily bear a direct relationship to cost. Reasonable charges for physician supervision were determined from current (1970) practices that were highly variable from facility to facility. A California study, for example, showed physician charges varying from $5.68 to $111.49 per dialysis session.[13] (We might note that this was still relatively early in the history of ESRD technology, and the functional role of the physician in ESRD care was still developing.) Although the government spent much time determining a reimbursement approach and rates, the final approach bore many similarities to one made by the National Kidney Foundation, which represented large segments of the medical community. Reimbursement for out-patient dialysis was to be based on a "reasonable charge" up to a screen (upper limit) for each dialysis treatment. The screen was set at $150 in cases where physicians are reimbursed by the facilities and routine lab tests were performed by the facilities. If physicians chose to be reimbursed a monthly capitation rate, the screen was set at $138. As of December 1980, physicians reimbursed under the "alternative method" provided three-fourths of all ESRD treatments.

When Exceptions Are the Rule: The Struggle with Case Mix

To accommodate those facilities whose costs have been unavoidably above the screen, a process was set up whereby facilities could apply for an exception to the reimbursement screen. In order to receive an exception, a facility had to submit current cost data and explanations for unavoidably high costs. By 1979, 29 percent of all dialysis facilities had received exceptions. By 1980, this figure had reached 34 percent. In 1979, 449 of the dialysis centers were independent (free-standing) units, and none of them had exceptions. Thus, almost 53 percent of the 526 hospital-based units were on a cost-based reimbursement system rather than being paid a capitation rate.[14]

The cost in dollars is difficult to estimate, as little data is collected on exceptions processed. One conservative estimate places the cost of exceptions granted by HCFA at a minimum of $71 million in 1979 alone.[15] Others, less conservative, have estimated this figure to be almost twice as high ($120 million).[16] These estimates are, of course, extremely crude, but they do demonstrate the magnitude of the impact of the exception process on ESRD program costs.

Free-standing facilities have virtually no exceptions, so it appears that the costs are related to characteristics of hospitals. Some believe that exceptions are often granted on the basis of poor data and the application of unclear and inconsistent criteria. Individual facility costs are compared with national and regional averages and, more often than not, exceptions are granted.

The government had little idea of how much to pay for dialysis. The screens set initially in 1972 were presented as representing the cost of treating the "average" ESRD patient. (Note: the average patient in 1972 was probably not as severe as the same patients are now.) "I suspect that we set the dialysis payment levels much too high in the beginning," said a former official in the program. "We really just picked them out of a hat."[17] No matter what is the actual relationship between resource utilization and cost, the screens suggest a different problem. If all facilities treating patients have similar resource requirements, then this is a fair, if overgenerous, rate structure. On the other hand, if different types of facilities have widely differing resource requirements, then some are overpaid and others are underpaid. The presence of a large number of profit-making dialysis facilities (nearly 40 percent), which together account for nearly $1 billion in federal payments from Medicare, compounds the problem.

New evidence suggested that there was a problem. A 1980 HCFA audit of facility reports of costs found that the median cost per treatment for hospital-based facilities ($135 per treatment) exceeded median costs for free-standing facilities ($108 per treatment) in the areas of labor, overhead, and supplies. Still, no one knew what these new data meant. They might indicate that the for-profit facilities were quite efficient and that hospitals were extremely inefficient. On the other hand, hospitals could have been treating sicker and more costly patients than the profit-making facilities were, a difference that would account for the cost differences. Millions of dollars in federal reimbursement hinged on the technical questions of who was treating whom at what costs. Congressional pressures for cost control would force HCFA to draw on the information from the audits to set reimbursement policy. It seemed that either hospitals or profit-making facilities were getting too much money. At stake was the now-popular notion of private-market efficiency in health services; did the facts bear out the promise?

Thrust and Parry: NMC Responds

Ten months after the opening salvo by Relman in the *NEJM*, the president (C. L. Hampers, M.D.) and vice-president (E. G. Lowrie, M.D.) of NMC countered. "The Success of Medicare's End-Stage Renal Disease Program: The Case for Profits and the Private Marketplace"—the title almost tells the story.[18] The text, however, displayed clearly the logic of the corporate approach to health policy and the article was intended to demonstrate generically "the case for profits":

> Some have cautioned that a new "medical-industrial complex," which could have an adverse effect on medical care, may be emerging . . . . The weight of evidence suggests, however, that these charges are highly inflated if not completely untrue. As we hope to show, the ESRD program has been highly successful in many ways, and there is a strong case to be made for the role of the profit incentive and the private marketplace—not only in the ESRD program but in the delivery of health care generally.[19]

Again, we see that ESRD is used as much for its symbolic value representing a "public problem" as for the actual issues grounded in patient care.

Lowrie and Hampers turn the "medical-industrial complex" argument on its head. For them, the medical-industrial complex is part of the solution, *not* part of the problem. "We should not fear 'the new medical-industrial complex.' Instead, we should learn to use it to its fullest potential to provide high-quality medical care efficiently."[20]

How is this so? Their argument seems straightforward but the assumptions are perplexing.

Here is a summary of the "case." First, the federal program is a success because it has recognized the efficiency of the private market. Because the government placed a cap on the price of dialysis ($138 per treatment in 1981), it created an incentive system ideally geared to market competition. The most efficient providers would deliver the most benefits. The government, however, hedged a bit. It paid hospitals a bit more through exemptions to the screen, an average of $159 per treatment (see Chapter 5 for a more complete discussion of reimbursement issues). As a result, and this is NMC's major point, hospitals receive a price subsidy. They get a higher payment and they do not pay taxes. On the other hand, profit-making centers pay taxes and are paid less by the government—obviously, the better buy for the taxpayers, reason Lowrie and Hampers.

Do hospitals treat sicker patients, thus incurring higher costs? Lowrie and Hampers assume that they do not. This is the cornerstone of the analysis, but their article addresses it only obliquely:

> One might argue that the example is contrived (which it is) and that hospitals do have higher costs, so that their profits are not as high as the example suggests. Perhaps, but the reimbursement rates are correct according to the HCFA, and for-profit facilities do pay taxes, thereby reducing net cost.[21]

A common rhetorical device is to downplay a problematic assumption and elevate a shadow issue to a prominent status in your argument. The shadow issue in the Lowrie and Hampers paper is an obscure discussion about price subsidies and the high costs of nonprofit organizations in general. The force of the shadow argument derives from the nondiscussion of the types of patients that hospitals actually treat. If hospitals do in fact treat sicker and more costly patients, the entire argument falls apart.

What did NMC gain from this presentation of the issues? In a prestigious medical journal it "proved" that for-profit facilities are responsible for cost control and nonprofits are wasteful, oversubsidized, and a burden to the taxpayer. The woeful performance of nonprofits, then, is the critical public problem. The authors suggested the elimination of both price and tax subsidies, proposing that all providers be paid the same. The public should not have to pay for higher prices for the same services. This is a boldly assertive but entirely unsubstantiated claim. It was countered in four strongly worded letters to the editor six months later, but the framework for debate had been defined by NMC.[22] Lowrie and Hampers chastised critics of the article for being naive and asserted that "available data and *economic theory* suggest contrary opinions."[23] Further, Lowrie and Hampers said that *they* recognized the "principles of economic utility," whereas their critics were economically unschooled.[24] Wrapped in the mantle of market rationality, NMC could now position itself as the cost-effective alternative in policy debates over federal reimbursement.

Facts and Fantasies: The Politics of Reimbursement

The government had to set some policy for a change in payment regardless of what was known about treatment costs. Congress had mandated that a change was in order. And so, revised reimbursement regulations for the ESRD program were proposed in February 1982. A proposed method for setting rates for dialysis services would establish "composite" rates for home and in-facility treatments that distinguish between hospital-based and independent facilities. Each facility would receive a certain rate per treatment, adjusted for geographic differences in the cost of labor. The average adjusted rate per treatment would be $128 for independent facilities and $132 for hospital-based facilities. What did all this mean?

In the first place, HCFA would pay different reimbursement rates to the hospital and free-standing facilities. Previous audits had shown a difference in costs between these types of facilities, and different payment levels seemed a logical extension of this "fact." But how equitable was the payment difference? Table 15 shows the net effect of the proposed rates compared with the audited costs of the two facilities. Hospitals would lose $6 per dialysis session whereas the free-standing facilities (90 percent profit-making) would *gain* $20 per dialysis treatment. Hospitals would lose, on average, $936 per patient per year (calculated at three treatments per week times fifty-two weeks). Free-standing facilities would gain $3,120 per patient per year. It seemed that the for-profits would be the big winners in this regulatory reshuffling and that the hospitals might have legitimate financial concerns. Equity, however, is in the eye of the beholder. The profit-making facilities were outraged at the proposed regula-

Table 15
Payment Rates: Hospitals versus Profit-making Facilities

Cost Estimate	Hospitals ($)	Free-Standing ($)
Audited costs	138	108
Proposed rates	132	128
Difference	(6)	20

Source: A. Plough, M. Shwartz, and S. Salem, "Greater Efficiency on Case-Mix Differences?: Fact vs. Fantasy in ESRD Reimbursement Policy," *Dialysis and Transplantation* 13 , Oct. 1984, p. 18.

tions. Dr. Hampers of NMC warned that the new rates would be discriminatory and would force his company to shut down 60 of its 160 clinics, which would force nearly 3,000 patients to find an alternative treatment setting. (Baxter Travenol, the large manufacturer of dialysis equipment, made a quick offer to buy the threatened clinics from NMC, which was refused.) Here we see a different assessment of the facts. Profit-making facilities considered the previous level of federal reimbursement as a starting point. These rates paid about $138 per dialysis to the free-standing facilities, so that the proposed regulations represented a potential loss of $10 per dialysis treatment ($1,560 per patient per year). For profit-making facilities, the difference between the "cost"-based analysis and the reimbursement-based estimates is almost $5,000 per patient per year.

Any manner of calculation, however, indicates that the hospitals are the losers in the composite-rate approach; the range of possible loss is from $3,640 to $936 per patient each year, depending on the cost assumptions.

NMC also raised the issue of patients' rights; the new rates would force patients to use less costly home dialysis, which was, in Hampers's opinion, unreasonable and potentially harmful. NMC supported a rally of 100 kidney patients at DHHS headquarters to protest "forced" home dialysis; it also filed suit against the government. This rhetoric scared kidney patients and their families, and it also received considerable press coverage.[25] HCFA ultimately felt the pressure.

Recalls an HCFA spokesman: "We got all kinds of letters from people who could barely write, saying, 'Don't kill my wife' or 'Don't let my son die.' They had been led to believe we were trying to force people off of dialysis. It was a horror show."[26]

The National Association of Patients on Hemodialysis and Transplantation, representing patients' interests in ESRD policy, claimed that more than 10,000 kidney patients would be affected by the change in regulation. These patients would be forced to move to quasi-experimental treatment modalities such as CAPD, which is possibly less costly to HCFA but potentially more costly to the patient in terms of increased risk of mortality and morbidity.[27]

The Healing Hand of the Market?

Implicit in this controversy over the facts and figures of dialysis reimbursement are a number of generic issues that are relevant to broader issues in public policy. One of these is the contrast between the hope attached to market fixes as a policy panacea and the actual performance of private firms engaged in the delivery of public welfare services. Remember that dialysis is a life-and-death service for the ESRD patient; the "consumer" cannot shop around, compare prices, and weigh the trade-offs. This is a dependency relationship of the most extreme kind. The government decided that all patients in need had a right to such treatment and that it was the responsibility of a federal program to act as a broker—certifying, paying for, and regulating the services for the entitled population. Clearly this is a large and complex task. If the "invisible hand" of the market could ease the burden of governmental responsibility without causing additional problems, it would lessen the bureaucratic implications of a major moral and financial commitment. The critically important question is whether that scenario is based in fact or in fantasy. What is the evidence (in the ESRD example) that fixed prices plus a mixed profit-making and nonprofit delivery system equal efficiency, not to mention equity? There was substantial controversy, confusion, and even acrimony surrounding this issue, but very little evidence.

The proposed regulations included much stricter controls on the exception process. HCFA hoped that many fewer facilities would require exceptions to their payment rate in the new dual-rate structure. They reasoned that hospitals and clinics would cut costs by training more patients to treat themselves at home. The "stick" in this proposition was reduced payment levels. The "carrot" was that providers would be paid the standard rates no matter where the patients were treated. The cheaper the per-patient costs, the greater the potential profit. Savings to the government might equal $300 million by 1985 if the incentive system worked as planned. Much of the regulatory burden, then, would shift to market forces. The government assumes that all facilities treat roughly similar types of patients (standard product), and it is up to the treatment facilities to prove otherwise. Exceptions would be considered only when a facility was able to provide convincing objective evidence that it had excessive costs attributable to an atypical patient mix, extraordinary circumstances (e.g., natural disasters), educational costs, or being an isolated essential facility.

The Question of Atypical Case Mix

Although HCFA gave four acceptable reasons for exceptions, it has not been so clear as to how actual determinations of cost differences due to these factors will be made.[28] Extraordinary circumstances, by their very nature, cannot all be itemized or predicted. The criteria for defining atypical patient mix are much less clear than in the other areas and, again, there is no indication of how these cost relationships will be determined. According to the proposed regulations, "any facility claiming to meet this criterion must demonstrate that its excess costs are not out of line with the standards of other facilities with a similar patient-mix."[29]

There are several problems with this approach to measuring atypical case mix. First, there is no clear definition of *typical* case mix. It is impossible to tell from available data what are the normal or average percentages of brittle diabetics or severe cancer cases in ESRD facilities. Second is the reliance on comparative data. Although improvements are being made in federal data collection systems, currently available federal data would not support an analysis of case mix on a facility-by-facility basis. Patient information is often missing or incomplete, and patient movement between facilities in and of itself is not reported. It is, therefore, up to a facility to measure independently its own case mix without federal definitions of what the concept really means.

Case-Mix Analysis in ESRD: An Approach to the Problem

Studies using the federal data base present conflicting results and suffer from two deficiencies that limit the generalizability of their findings.[30] First, comorbidity characteristics could not be included as they are not routinely reported. Comorbidity is often as important a factor as primary diagnosis when approaching case-mix issues in an area of chronic illness.[31] Second, the federal data, especially the clinical information for particular patients, is inadequate because of incomplete reporting practices. In some states only 50 percent of facilities even report data to the government. Even those facilities that do report will have, on average, 40 percent of the variables missing.[32]

Clearly, case-mix differences are a key to the question of who is treating whom and allows an empirical linkage to the issue of cost comparison between hospitals and profit-making facilities. The linchpin of NMC's claim of greater efficiency is that their patients are just like patients treated in hospitals. In fact, Hampers and Lowrie suggest that patients in profit-making facilities are *more* difficult to treat than hospital-based patients.[33] This was also the basis for a lawsuit against the proposed changes in payment levels; no study has shown that there are case-mix differences between hospitals and profit-making facilities. In NMC's opinion, therefore, the regulations are arbitrary and unfair.

Corporate Pressure and the Politics of Research: "This Study Will Hurt Us"

The tone and concerns of the Lowrie letter should now be more understandable. Millions of dollars in potential Medicare reimbursement could be affected if the contention that there are no case-mix differences was questioned by a detailed and representative study. Proposed federal regulations assumed some degree of increased severity in hospital-based ESRD patients but had no real data to back up even this mild assumption. Lowrie and Hampers had published two studies that suggested the great efficiency of the profit-making facilities. A lawsuit based on these "facts" challenged the federal government to substantiate proposed changes in payment policies. The parameters for the battle were set and the evidence seemed clear.

For three years a research group I headed examined the issue of case mix in ESRD treatment facilities using a data base created from the Michigan Kidney Registry.[34] Using patient characteristics and information on survival, we were able to classify patients into groups according to their relative severity and to use these groups to examine case mix across types of ESRD treatment facilities. Here is how we looked at the problem.

Patients were first assigned a diagnostic code based on their most severe primary renal diagnosis or comorbid condition. Using multiple-regression techniques, we determined the relationship of these diagnostic variables, age, and race to patient survival. Based on the regression equation, patients were assigned scores that represented their relative risk of survival, or probability of death. Patients were then combined into five severity groups, the highest having the greatest risk of dying. In order to measure case mix, we examined the distribution of these severity groups within different types of ESRD treatment facilities. This analysis was conducted twice, the first time using one-year survival as the dependent variable, the second time using survival over the course of treatment. The first of these allowed us to examine case mix defined by short-term risk: how diagnosis, age, and race were related to survival over the first year of treatment. The second model using length of survival allowed us to estimate the risk of death over the entire course of treatment and to examine case mix using a long-term definition of risk.

Our findings indicated that hospital-based facilities had a significantly larger percentage of patients in the higher risk groups than did free-standing profit-making facilities, that is, a more severe case mix (Table 16). This held true using both the long- and short-term risk models, the latter having a high level of statistical significance. A

Table 16
Percentage of Patients in Various Severity Groups
According to Facility Type

Facility Comparison	*Severity Group**					*p Value*
	1	*2*	*3*	*4*	*5*	
Logistic						
Hospital-based	20	21	21	20	19	
(N = 3,135)						0.02
Free-standing	24	26	17	16	17	
(N = 307)						
Proportional hazard						
Hospital-based	19	20	20	21	20	
(N = 3,135)						0.07
Free-standing	21	24	22	16	17	
(N = 307)						

*Groups range from 1, least severe, to 5, most severe.

more detailed discussion of the methodology and findings can be found in the Appendix. This study strongly supported the view that measurable case-mix differences do exist between individual ESRD treatment facilities. The manuscript was submitted to the *New England Journal of Medicine* in May 1983.

NMC's senior vice-president, E. G. Lowrie, seemed greatly perturbed by this study. He suggested in a telephone call to me that I should get a lawyer because his counsel suggested that my study raised serious problems far beyond a "freedom of speech issue." He wondered why I chose to send the paper to the *NEJM* and not the *American Journal of Statistics*, where publication of the findings would concern him much less. Dr. Lowrie assured me that he would investigate the matter and take the appropriate remedies.

On May 10 Lowrie sent a letter to HCFA, which had funded my current study and was considering a new grant application in a related area. He enclosed the letter to me (quoted at the beginning of the chapter) and a cover letter to the director of the Office of Research and Demonstrations, from which I take the following quotations:

I enclose a letter to Dr. Alonzo Plough describing my concerns. The redundant nature of the analysis sadly distorts its interpretation. If, for example, there were more blond-haired, blue-eyed individuals treated by hospitals, and if hair color and eye color were included as potential risk factors in the primary analysis, Dr. Plough may well have found that blond hair and blue eyes correlate with mortality. He would then have discovered that hospitals treat more blond-haired, blue-eyed individuals and thus would conclude that they treat a more severe case mix. Additional grant monies would then be awarded to determine whether or not it costs more to treat blond-haired, blue-eyed patients, and so it goes.

I hate to reduce my objections to this ridiculous example; however, it does illustrate nicely how the structural logic of the analysis distorts the facts. The main issue is reduced survival in hospitals and not the case mix as this study mistakenly implies.

Only two days later (12 May 1983) Dr. Lowrie sent another letter to HCFA. In this missive he raised the "quality of care" issue and stated:

Essentially, the treatment prescription may well affect the morbidity and mortality which patients experience. Our thesis is that

Dr. Plough failed to account for treatment quality in his analysis. We believe that his data suggests that treatment was inferior in hospital-based facilities.

I enclose several articles which were published in the April issue of *Kidney International* describing the results of the National Cooperative Dialysis Study. I believe the enclosed summarize the essence of the material.

Lowrie was the lead investigator in the National Cooperative Dialysis (NCD) study.

On 21 June 1983 Dr. Lowrie wrote again, this time sending to HCFA a detailed statistical review (five pages, single spaced) of our study. From this it became clear that he was working from a very early first draft and had not seen the final study. How he got hold of those drafts is unclear. The "outside" statistical evaluator of this review had worked under Lowrie in the NCD study. Surprisingly, her findings replicated Lowrie's initial concerns about our findings. We had not found case-mix differences but had really demonstrated that nonprofit hospitals were actually killing off ESRD patients at a statistically significant rate.

The letter campaign attempted to ridicule and trivialize our study. Further, as Dr. Lowrie knew that I had a grant application pending at HCFA, he wished to establish the fruitlessness of awarding any future monies to support such "distorted" research. These letters were the only evidence of pressures brought to bear on HCFA concerning my research, but there was other activity. However, it was the hard-to-document use of power by a corporation that has considerable resources and strong political connections within the Reagan administration.

There was another thrust to this effort to undermine the findings on case-mix differences: an attack at the potential source of publication. The *NEJM* received at least three letters from the prolific Dr. Lowrie presenting a similar picture of the research on case-mix differences. One of these was the statistical review sent to HCFA with a cover letter to Dr. Relman, editor of the journal. In this letter, Dr. Lowrie suggested that the *NEJM* might not be capable of reviewing my manuscript.

As noted, physician reviewers are not likely to be sufficiently sophisticated to determine the inadequacies of the case mix analysis. In addition, some statisticians who have no knowledge of

ESRD treatment may not be able to apply their conceptual statistical knowledge to the ESRD environment. We chose Dr. Laird because she has combined expertise in both areas.

To sum up this unusual episode, Dr. Lowrie put significant energy into a concerted four- or five-month effort to crush both the publication of a completed study and the funding of future research on case-mix differences. What was the result of these efforts? Mixed. The manuscript was published in the *NEJM*. The influence of the NMC pressure, however, resulted in an overly cautious (even defensive) tone in the editing of the final manuscript. In an article in *Barron's*, Dr. Relman said the study provoked an "intense" and "unusual" lobbying campaign by a major corporate owner of kidney dialysis centers to block its publication.[35] Our $900,000 grant to HCFA was not funded in spite of strong support from officials within the federal program. It is impossible to gauge the influence of the NMC activities on this decision. Clearly, the letters had created a negative environment around the application within the agency. The nature of power, particularly the diffuse power of a corporation, however, is difficult to track.

We must understand the true cost of patient treatment if we are to develop effective and equitable rates of reimbursement. The potential role of case mix in the generation of facility costs is of considerable importance to policy decisions in this area. If systematic variation in case mix by type of facility is evident throughout the system, then reimbursement policies that do not consider case mix are probably not equitable. The effect of current flat-rate reimbursement policies would be to overpay facilities that characteristically treat a less severe case mix and underpay those that treat a more severe case mix.

Is equity a concern in the calculus of Reagan's health policy? For that matter, is empirical data that important to current policy makers? The ideology of market efficiency fuels itself. As the profit-making sector becomes increasingly involved in the delivery of health services, research on the characteristics of these firms becomes more than just scientific interest. It potentially influences the corporate bottom line. At least, this is NMC's assumption. The scientific agenda and the ideological agenda become blurred. The real battle is over the guiding framework for federal health policy: Equity or efficiency? Public welfare or private profit? These are the choices. Perhaps these are not, ultimately, dichotomies, and policies can allow for both concerns to be advanced. Recent federal policies, however, indicate that efficiency and profits are dominant influences. There is limited recognition of complex issues concerning values that underlie the "objective" pursuit of these outcomes.

EPILOGUE

Hope in the New Machine: Medical Ritual and Market Mythology

What is the pattern that connects the chapters of this book? We have moved from the public perception of a technological wonder, through a more direct experience with life and death in the clinic, and finally to a public battle over profits and efficiency. All of these stories concern the experience of medical technology but in varied settings and with different emphasis. The common thread is dependency: each chapter considers a particular type of dependent relationship with medical technology.

Within the cognitive order of the clinic we see a dependency fueled by a collective notion of techno-science, a group of clinical scientists who embody their expertise in a technological form. They depend on technical fixes to establish professional legitimacy. Professional success seems gauged by an effective public demonstration of mastery over a *technical body of knowledge* that can effectively (or at least rhetorically) substitute for the unmanageable social body of a diverse group of patients. The cognitive order of the clinic depends on a way of knowing in which broad uncertainties and contingencies are reformed within a technical corpus. Like Margaret Mead's Samoan adolescents, the clinicians experienced a "coming of age" when the youthful technique of dialysis matured and proliferated.

Although physicians may dispute the relative merit of new techniques, they also reduce the range of "acceptable" analysis. The variable and socially embedded patient becomes, too often, of adjunct concern. Of course, studies of survival and rehabilitation are proxies for a concern with the patient but in an aggregate, statistical form. These groupings are easily amendable to very narrow measures, such as length of survival (instead of quality of life) or employment (as a substitute for social integration).

In the treatment setting itself, the problematic assumptions of clinical theory come home to roost. Practitioners depend on the logic of the technical body but are forced to experience the wide-ranging social contingencies of chance, luck, hope, fear, and trust. Their struggle to define success is a dialectical journey between the assumptions of technical theory and the experiential conditions of life, death, and uncertainty.

Medical-social research gropes for a framework to synthesize clinical expectations and the social conditions of the experience of living and dying within a technology. It is no surprise that clinical theory dominates this viewpoint and that social factors are merely substitute variables in the medical equation. The social frame is a medical gaze in spite of itself.[1]

The uplifting and optimistic story within all of this is that patients and practitioners struggle to reinterpret their own experience and endure in spite of the various professional frames. Some practitioners even learn from uncertainty rather than simply resisting it. "Successful" patients learn that hope must be placed primarily in their own will to endure and only secondarily in the promises of the technical body. The will to endure, however, must emerge through a complex social potential and against biological limitations. Social conditions like income, social support, or education as well as the biology of the disease exert their own forces. Through understanding the dynamics of experience, we see clinical problems in more human terms.

A "public" problem emerges from the experience of medical technology: it is very expensive. Here we see another level of dependency, where the technology "needs" a large amount of capital to function. The capital requirements of dialysis and transplantation go beyond the usual resource capacities of individuals or families. Thus, the technology becomes a social welfare issue. In the public realm certain internal contradictions of medical technology become clear: inequalities in access and the class-based judgments that occur when tragic choices must be made. These contradictions threaten to reveal all too explicitly that life is not fair. Race, money, status, and productivity become de facto assessments of worth and influence one's chances for life. Of course, these factors always influence life expectancy. Any perusal of U.S. mortality rates comparing blacks with whites, or poor with nonpoor, indicates the same thing. But there is an important political distinction between the aggregate demonstration that inequality kills and the highly visible individual examples of the same social fact.

The government depends on regulation and categorical entitlements to focus attention away from the broader issues of inequality. It defines the equity dilemma as a management problem of paying for one obvious example of a specific need, an extreme medical technology. This is an apparently simple but extremely complex form of dependency. The rhetoric of federal involvement seems straightforward: accept the clinical definition of the problem, assume a "neutral" role toward the profit-nonprofit conundrum, and demand "efficiency" from the providers. If the profit-making facilities are more efficient than the nonprofits, so be it. The imperative is to save money.

The complexities introduced by these simple assumptions are profound. They combine the unchallenged assumptions of clinical theory and the ideal of market efficiency into a bureaucratic notion of cost effectiveness. As the discussion of the rapid growth of the dialysis industry (Chapter 6) and the dynamics of the disease market (Chapter 7) indicate, the assumptions break down in practice. The ideal of market efficiency is not substantiated. Segmenting patients by severity characteristics and selectively treating a very high proportion of those who are less sick may be cost-effective to the firm but it is not to the public payer. It represents an efficient business practice (like economies of scale or vertical integration) but does not enhance the public good. Further, the effects of these practices on the quality of life of kidney patients is questionable, although this is difficult to measure except at the extremes.

Medical technology and the market metaphor provide a powerful influence on the experience of illness. This is highlighted in the case of catastrophic illnesses requiring extreme technical interventions but is a characteristic of the health care system as a whole. Technology and the market have proven to be the Scylla and Charybdis of health care policy in the United States. Yet both areas are highly resistant to critical scrutiny because they embody powerful symbolic categories: "objective" science and the "logic" of rational individualism. These two ideological frames operate beyond the sphere of medicine and provide the root metaphors for Western society. The objectivity of science and the logic of the market are key organizing principles of power and order.[2]

Within the culture of medicine, prestige and income are directly related to the dependency of practice on symbols of technical expertise. In fact, the most financially lucrative medical practices (such as pathology and radiology) are entirely focused on technique and are removed from social interaction with a complex, living patient. Pediatrics and public health, more firmly grounded in the social aspects of illness, are at the bottom rung of medical status and prestige.

The case of ESRD describes the relationship between knowledge, power, professional interest, and human needs within the culture of medicine. It is a particularly dramatic example but not an unrepresentative one. The social history of this medical technology moves quickly from promising experiment to legitimate therapy to federally funded program and finally to return on equity discussed in the corporate boardrooms. This is a compressed history that parallels the development of American medicine during the last fifty years.[3]

ESRD continues to play a key symbolic role in U.S. health policy. This was most clearly demonstrated in a 1984 book by Henry J. Aaron and William B. Schwartz, *The Painful Prescription: Rationing Hospital Care*. In this highly influential book (both in the professional world and in the mass media) the authors argue that Americans will be forced to limit or ration medical care because of the increasing costs of hospital care and in particular new medical technologies. Dialysis and kidney transplantation provide the lead example in their chapter entitled "Matters of Life and Death." Can we afford such life-saving but expensive medical miracles? Aaron and Schwartz compared the rate of treatment for ESRD in Great Britain with that found in the United States and, like many previous researchers, found that the British rate is less than half the U.S. rate.

How do we interpret this striking difference? In Britain treatment is obviously denied to particular categories of patients but through a fuzzy set of implicit criteria (age, comorbidity, "social worth"). While there is considerable controversy as to exactly how this rationing activity operates in the context of individual decisions by doctors to deny treatment, the process seems rooted in the general resource constraints of the British national health service. How does this comparative example inform our analysis of the situation in the United States? I believe that it adds relatively little to our under-

standing of the culture of medical technology in America. Our
approach to the organization of medical care has always differed from
the British model, both in governmental policies and the social
context of patient care. The difference in dialysis rates, given the
clinical nature and the costs of ESRD, would be expected. The far
more interesting question is why this example becomes the focus of
so many professional and mass media discussions of U.S. ESRD
policy. This reflects, I would argue, a tendency to establish a public
moral debate over the denial of a specific "life-extending" technology
to an identified dying person. Since the early 1950s Americans have
been conditioned to expect that science and government will develop
medical miracles to save us from dread diseases and that there is a
"right" of access to these procedures once they have crossed the
threshold from experiment to therapy. The British counter-example
is often used to demonstrate that the United States has developed an
approach to the allocation of medical miracles that avoids public-level
ethical conflicts of choosing who lives and who dies. There is an
implicit message of moral superiority in this discourse that is usually
tempered only by the recognition that our approach costs too much.
This is just another example of the technological imperative argument consistent with the culture of medicine. The social logic of
rationing intensifies the focus on medical technology, employs only
surface models of technology assessment to discuss costs and effectiveness, and leaves unquestioned the cultural and political forces
that I have argued are essential to understanding our experience with
extreme medical technologies.

What about the artificial heart and the flurry of activity in organ
transplantation that has occurred since Barney Clark became indel-
ibly etched in the public consciousness as the symbol of the new
frontier in medical technology? It goes far beyond the scope of this
book to detail the latest example of our desperate hope in new
life-extending machines. I believe that the public drama surrounding
the artificial heart—the intense media attention, the role of a profit-
making corporation in the marketing of the technique, the extension
of the therapeutic applications, and the form of the ethical dialogue
surrounding this technique—are an extension of the issues raised in
the ESRD example. The more general public focus on organ transplantation and the rapid movement of both the federal government
and the states to accommodate the growth of these extreme medical
technologies also echo the history of ESRD. This is but another

chapter in a continuing story of the culture and politics of medical technology in America.

Yet we do not seem to learn from past experiences in health policy. There are many lessons from the end-stage renal disease program but conventional readings seem to focus on the surface phenomenon: resource allocation, decision making, cost containment, organ procurement programs, and the like. There is a pattern that connects the myriad of concerns in ESRD and it is as important to understand and learn from this pattern as it is to focus on clinical or bureaucratic puzzle-solving.

One thought seems to emerge from the various texts; we are all linked to technology and in many ways are machine-dependent. It is characteristic of American society

that technical forms do, to a large extent, shape the basic pattern and content of human activity in our time. Thus, politics becomes (among other things) an active encounter with the specific forms and processes contained in technology.

. . . that *technology is itself a political phenomenon*. A crucial turning point comes when one is able to acknowledge that modern technics, much more than politics as conventionally understood, now legislates the conditions of human existence. New technologies are institutional structures within an evolving constitution that gives shape to a new polity, the technopolis in which we do increasingly live. For the most part, this constitution still evolves with little public scrutiny or debate. Shielded by the conviction that technology is neutral and tool-like, a whole new order is built—piecemeal, step by step, with the parts and pieces linked together in novel ways—without the slightest public awareness or opportunity to dispute the character of the changes underway. It is somnambulism (rather than determinism) that characterizes technological politics—on the left, right, and center equally.[4]

Although the connections are not as obvious as in the case of the ESRD patient, we share the same root metaphor of survival and struggle within a similar dialectical relationship with expertise. The major differences are in the scale of dependency and the visibility of the ties that bind us to hope in the next new machine.

Appendix

Much of Chapter 7 draws on a large data base from the Michigan Kidney Registry that includes all ESRD patients starting treatment in the state over a nine-year period. The methodology used in examining the data base related patient characteristics and risk of mortality in ESRD by developing *severity groupings*—clusters of patients of similar risk but different clinical characteristics. The first step in doing this was to develop a reliable model to define patients' illness severity. First a model was developed and tested that quantified the variables related to survival and their relative effects. Based on this model risk groups were formed that could be used to analyze case mix in ESRD treatment.

The population of Michigan is very diverse, both geographically and socio-economically. There is a large nonwhite population and clearly distinguishable urban and rural areas. Michigan's ESRD population is in some important ways representative of the nation as a whole. Thirteen percent of all ESRD patients in Michigan are on home dialysis (U.S. mean is 13.1 percent), and the transplantation rate per million is 20 in Michigan compared to a national rate of 19.4.

The Michigan Kidney Registry (MKR) collects data on all ESRD patients under treatment by dialysis or transplantation in the State of Michigan. All ESRD treatment facilities in Michigan routinely report information to the Registry. In addition Registry personnel audit facilities once or twice a year to verify the completeness and accuracy of data reported. Information contained in the Registry includes socio-demographic characteristics, primary diagnosis, initial co-morbidity (comorbidity present at the start of ESRD treatment), treatment modality, and modality changes.

The data base constructed from the Registry contained 4,842 patients who began ESRD treatment between January 1973 and September 1981 at one of thirty-five Michigan ESRD treatment facilities. Of this group, patients beginning treatment prior to 1973 and the implementation of Section 2991 of the Social Security Act Amendments were excluded since, due to much stricter admissions criteria, they constitute a clinically different population. Patients at Veterans Administration hospitals and ESRD treatment facilities in Michigan's Upper Peninsula were also excluded from the analysis: VA patients are not relevant to a study of facility placement, since they are treated mostly in the VA hospitals, and, due to geographic location, facilities in the Upper Peninsula interact more closely with the ESRD network in Minnesota. These exclusions plus those due to missing (unreported) data and incomplete reporting reduced the sample to 4,451 patients.

Development of Severity Groups through Survival Analysis: Methods

The risk of death was estimated for each patient according to age, race, primary renal diagnosis, and comorbid conditions. Based on a risk score assigned to each patient, patients were grouped into five mutually exclusive severity groups. We then compared the distribution of these severity groups between hospital-based and free-standing facilities.

Risk of death was defined as the relative risk of death over the entire course of treatment. Relative risk of death over the course of treatment was estimated with the proportional hazard model. We used this model to estimate the risk of death associated with particular patient characteristics. The age variable associated with each patient was one of eight ten-year groupings. Race was defined as a dischotomous variable, white/nonwhite. Nearly 95 percent of the nonwhite patients in the sample were black.

A multistage procedure was used to develop the diagnostic variables. First, based on studies of ESRD patient survival and interviews with a sample of nephrologists, the extensive range of diagnostic conditions present in the MKR data base (over 200) was collapsed into eight primary renal and fourteen comorbid diagnostic categories. Conditions were combined that seemed meaningfully related to survival or formed clinically coherent groups. Further, preliminary analysis showed similar survival characteristics for patients with a given disease (for example, hypertension), whether the disease was reported as a primary renal diagnosis causing ESRD (nephrosclerosis) or as a comorbid condition (elevated blood pressure). Accordingly, all primary renal and comorbid diagnoses were combined, resulting in the following categories: cancer, diabetes mellitus, social/behavioral, heart disease, vascular disease, pulmonary disease, collagen disease, chronic glomerulonephritis, chronic interstitial nephritis, polycystic kidney disease, and "other" primary diagnosis.

Cox's Proportional Hazard

To identify the effect of prognostic variables on survival, we used Cox's proportional hazard model.

Let t_1 = survival of the ith patient and X_{i1}, $X_{i2} \ldots _{ip}$ be prognostic variables associated with the ith patient. We are interested in identifying a relationship between t_1, or a function of t_1, $g(t_1)$, and the p prognostic variables of the form:

$$g(t_1) = f(X_{i1}, X_{i2}, \ldots X_{ipi})$$

Ordinary multiple regression methods cannot be used for this problem because of the presence of censored data, which arise because some subjects are likely to be alive at the time of data collection. We will not know the survival time of these patients, only that they did not die in the period of time during which they were followed. To handle censored data using regression-type approaches, the assumption of proportional hazard functions is usually made. The most widely used model incorporating this assumption, Cox's proportional hazard model,[1] is a general nonparametric model appropriate for the analysis of survival data with and without censoring.

To explain Cox's model it is necessary to define *hazard function*. A hazard function is the probability that someone dies in a small interval of time, given that he or she survives to the beginning of that interval. In the proportional hazard model, hazard rates are used as dependent variables. Let $h_i t$ = hazard rate for the ith patient at time t, and let $X_{i1}, X_{i2}, \ldots X_{ip}$ be the value of p prognostic variables for the ith person. The proportional hazard model hypothesis is:

$$h_i(t) = h_o(t) \exp (\Sigma b_j X_{ji})$$

where $h_o(t)$ is the hazard function of some underlying arbitrary survival distribution when all p prognostic variables equal zero. Both sides of this equation are divided by $h_o(t)$; then the ratio $h_i(t)/h_o(t)$, which can be thought of as the relative risk of the ith person, is assumed to be constant over time. The log of the relative risk is assumed to be a linear function of the prognostic variables. For this analysis $h_i(t)/h_o(t)$ is the grouping variable.

Refinement of Model

Since patients in this data base are often classified as having multiple conditions, the coefficients determined from the initial analysis were difficult to interpret. The coefficient for a given diagnosis represented the average relative risk (of death) for all patients reporting that condition, many of whom also had other conditions present. There was no clear way to disentangle these interaction effects. This was especially problematic for a condition such as hypertension where most of the patients also presented more serious conditions. It was also unclear what baseline risk was being evaluated against.

These problems were approached in the following manner. First, using the coefficients from one of the initial regression models, the conditions were ranked in order of severity (higher relative risk = more severe). These rankings were generally consistent with clinical opinion. Every patient was assigned to one category based on the *most* severe condition present (Table 17). Added to the preliminary model were variables for two-way interactions. If patients had more than one condition, they were placed in a group for only the most "severe" interaction. In this way a model was developed based on mutually exclusive diagnostic categories. The coefficient for a single disease represented patients presenting with that disease only and no other conditions. The interaction variables represented patients for whom the two specified diseases were the most severe two conditions present. Attempts to investigate the interaction of more than two conditions revealed numbers too small for valid analysis.

There was little improvement in the goodness of fit of the model when the interaction terms were included. To simplify the application of the model and its interpretation, each patient was coded only for the most severe single condition in the final model.

An attempt was made to include a variable to describe "good

Table 17
Rank Order of Diagnostic Groups
from Highest to Lowest Severity

Group	No.
Cancer	74
Collagen disease	130
Diabetes	1,030
Social/behavioral	83
Cerebrovascular disease	44
Heart disease	243
Pulmonary disease	31
Hypertension	1,297
Other primary diagnosis	315
Chronic interstitial nephritis	218
Chronic glomerulonephritis	505
Polycystic kidney disease	0

health" or relative low risk by examining patient suitability for transplantation. Although the variable "candidate for transplant" is reported to the Registry, a low correlation was found between patients reported as candidates and those actually transplanted. This variable was not reliable enough to be included in the analysis. A variable was then created that included all patients who had ever been transplanted. This, however, confounded the analysis since the same characteristics related to survival may also be related to tranplantation, which in turn may affect survival.

The effect of age on survival independent of comorbidity was examined by including eight age variables in the final model. This allowed us to see the differential effect of age by ten-year age groups (the oldest group included ages 70–90 due to small numbers). Previous research suggests that relative risk increases exponentially with each additional ten years of age.[2]

In the preliminary model the coefficient for the age and diagnostic variables described the proportional hazard, or risk of death, compared to a group with age of 0 and no comorbidity whatsoever. This group consisted of patients in the 41–50-year-old age group, white, and reporting only chronic glomerulonephritis. The age group was chosen based on the mean sample age of 48. The disease classification was chosen since it is considered to be one of the less complicated subgroups of ESRD patients.

Race was included in the model as a bivariate function (white/nonwhite) as a third descriptive category.

The Final Proportional Hazard Model

The selected race, diagnostic, and age variables were included in a multiple regression using Cox's proportional hazard model. The results of this analysis are presented in Table 18. (A negative coefficient indicates a positive relationship to survival.)

The statistically significant coefficients represent the increased (or decreased) risk of death compared to a baseline patient who is white and aged 41–50 with chronic glomerulonephritis. Unlike the current research literature, where nonwhite patients appear to have both a higher incidence of ESRD disease and, in some studies, a poorer overall survival outcome than whites, in our model the proportional hazard model shows no significant difference between nonwhites and

Table 18
Cox's Proportional Hazard Model

Variable	Coefficient	Significance
Race	.0074	.8819
Age 0–10*	− 1.322	.0017
Age 11–20†	− 1.0524	.0000
Age 21–30†	− .5293	.0000
Age 31–40†	− .3286	.0004
Age 41–50	0	baseline
Age 51–60†	.2791	.0000
Age 61–70†	.4722	.0000
Age 71–90†	.8133	.0000
Cancer†	.9622	.0000
Collagen disease†	.9095	.0000
Diabetes†	.6386	.0000
Social/behavioral†	.5176	.0038
Cerebrovascular disease†	.5345	.0096
Heart disease*	.2563	.0202
Lung disease	.3543	.1822
Hypertension	.1228	.1127
Chronic interstitial nephritis	.1986	.0613
Chronic glomerulonephritis	0	baseline
Other primary diagnosis†	.5566	.0000

*p (≤) .05.
†p (≤) .005.

whites in terms of survival when age and comorbidity are controlled. The age variables are all significant in the expected directions with the largest coefficients belonging to the groups farthest from the baseline age group; this is consistent with previous studies showing that increasing age decreases the probability of survival. The coefficients for cancer, collagen disease, diabetes, social, heart, cardiovascular disease, and other primary diagnosis are all significant; these conditions are found to increase relative risk compared to the baseline. Pulmonary disease is also found to be associated with a higher risk of death, but the coefficient is not statistically significant. Hypertension in this model is not associated with an increased or decreased risk of death compared to the baseline group.

Formulation of Risk Clusters

To interpret the proportional hazard model in terms of risk, we know that the log of relative risk is a linear function of the independent variables. Therefore, to determine the relative risk attached to each variable we calculate $e^{B_i X_i}$, where $B_i X_i$ = the coefficient for an independent variable. Table 19 presents the relative risk attached to each statistically significant variable in the model.

Table 19
Calculation of Relative Risk

Variable	Coefficient $(B_i X_i)$	Rel. Risk $(e^{B_i X_i})$
Age 0–10	1.1322	.32
Age 11–20	− 1.0524	.35
Age 21–30	− .5293	.59
Age 31–40	− .3286	.72
Age 41–50	0	1.00
Age 51–60	.2791	1.32
Age 61–70	.4722	1.604
Age 71–90	.8133	2.26
Cancer	.9622	2.62
Collagen disease	.9095	2.48
Diabetes	.6386	1.89
Social/behavioral	.5176	1.68
Cerebrovascular disease	.5345	1.72
Heart disease	.2563	1.29
Interstitial nephritis	.1986	1.220
Other primary diagnosis	.5566	1.75

Based on the proportional hazard model we can calculate the relative risk for any individual patient:

$$RR = e^{B_i X_i}.$$

Given the manner in which the data are coded, a patient will have at least a significant age coefficient and at most a significant age coefficient and one significant diagnostic coefficient, indicating the presence of one of the conditions determined by the proportional hazard model to be significantly related to relative risk. The resulting risk figure is the same as would be calculated by multiplying the age risk factor by the diagnostic risk factor. For example, a patient aged 31–40 (.65) with diabetes (1.66) would have a relative risk value of 1.08 (.65 × 1.66). Figure 5 shows the distribution of relative risk in this population.

Five mutually exclusive risk groups were formed, each containing approximately 20 percent of the sample population. Table 20 presents the risk ranges and sizes of these subsamples.

Each age × diagnosis combination places a patient in one of these five groups. Table 21 presents the patient characteristic combinations by risk group. "No significant morbidity" refers to those patients who have none of the diagnostic characteristics found to be statistically significant and whose relative risk is increased by only the age effect.

Testing the Proportional Hazard Model

To assess the validity of the proportional hazard assumption[3] suggests plotting the log of the cumulative hazard function against time.

Table 20
Relative Risk Groups—Proportional Hazard Model

Risk Group	Range	N	Weighted Average Risk	Percent
1	0–.72	890	.60	20.0
2	.73–1.29	758	1.05	17.1
3	1.30–1.60	1043	1.44	23.4
4	1.61–2.48	839	2.00	18.8
5	2.49+	921	3.09	20.7

Figure 5
Distribution of Relative Risk in the Proportional Hazard Model

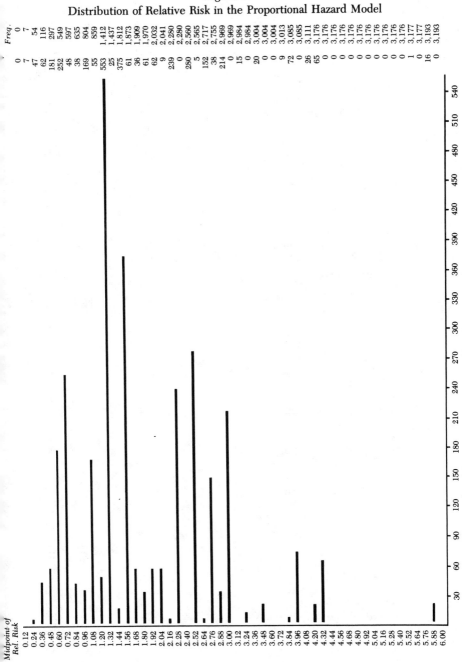

Freq.	
0	0
7	7
54	47
116	62
297	181
549	252
597	48
635	38
804	169
859	55
1,412	553
1,437	25
1,812	375
1,873	61
1,909	36
1,970	61
2,032	62
2,041	9
2,280	239
2,280	0
2,560	280
2,565	5
2,717	152
2,755	38
2,969	214
2,969	0
2,984	15
2,984	0
3,004	20
3,004	0
3,004	0
3,013	9
3,085	72
3,085	0
3,111	26
3,176	65
3,176	0
3,176	0
3,176	0
3,176	0
3,176	0
3,176	0
3,176	0
3,176	0
3,177	1
3,193	16
3,193	0

Midpoint of Rel. Risk: 0.12, 0.24, 0.36, 0.48, 0.60, 0.72, 0.84, 0.96, 1.08, 1.20, 1.32, 1.44, 1.56, 1.68, 1.80, 1.92, 2.04, 2.16, 2.28, 2.40, 2.52, 2.64, 2.76, 2.88, 3.00, 3.12, 3.24, 3.36, 3.48, 3.60, 3.72, 3.84, 3.96, 4.08, 4.20, 4.32, 4.44, 4.56, 4.68, 4.80, 4.92, 5.04, 5.16, 5.28, 5.40, 5.52, 5.64, 5.76, 5.88, 6.00

Axis: 30, 60, 90, 120, 150, 180, 210, 240, 270, 300, 330, 360, 390, 420, 450, 480, 510, 540

Table 21
Risk Groups—Proportional Hazard Model

Risk Group	RR	N
Risk Group 1 (0–.72)		
Age 0–10, no sig. morbidity	.32	19
Age 0–10, interstitial nephr.	.39	2
Age 0–10, heart disease	.42	5
Age 0–10, social	.54	1
Age 0–10, other primary	.56	21
Age 0–10, diabetes	.61	1
Age 11–20, no sig. morbidity	.35	109
Age 11–20, interstitial nephr.	.43	33
Age 11–20, heart disease	.45	6
Age 11–20, social	.59	4
Age 11–20, cv	.60	1
Age 11–20, other primary	.61	54
Age 11–20, diabetes	.66	7
Age 21–30, no sig. morbidity	.59	267
Age 21–30, interstitial nephr.	.72	43
Age 31–40, no. sig. morbidity	.72	317
Total		890
Risk Group 2 (.73–1.29)		
Age 11–20, collagen disease	.87	19
Age 21–30, heart disease	.76	14
Age 21–30, social	.99	16
Age 21–30, cv	1.01	51
Age 21–30, other primary	1.03	1
Age 21–30, diabetes	1.12	118
Age 31–40, interstitial nephr.	.88	29
Age 31–40, heart disease	.93	21
Age 31–40, social	1.21	16
Age 31–40, cv	1.23	1
Age 31–40, other primary	1.26	38
Age 41–50, no sig. morbidity	1.00	363
Age 41–50, interstitial nephr.	1.22	44
Age 41–50, heart disease	1.29	27
Total		758
Risk Group 3 (1.30–1.60)		
Age 21–30, collagen disease	1.46	25
Age 31–40, diabetes	1.36	156
Age 51–60, no sig. morbidity	1.33	466
Age 61–70, no sig. morbidity	1.60	396
Total		1043

Table 21 *(Continued)*

Risk Group	RR	N
Risk Group 4 (1.61–2.48)		
Age 31–40, collagen disease	1.79	36
Age 31–40, cancer	1.88	1
Age 41–50, social	1.68	24
Age 41–50, cardiovascular	1.71	4
Age 41–50, other primary	1.75	53
Age 41–50, collagen disease	2.48	21
Age 41–50, diabetes	1.89	147
Age 51–60, interstitial nephr.	1.63	78
Age 51–60, heart disease	1.72	61
Age 51–60, social	2.24	9
Age 51–60, cardiovascular	2.26	17
Age 51–60, other primary	2.32	85
Age 61–70, interstitial nephr.	1.96	60
Age 61–70, heart disease	2.07	62
Age 71–90, no sig. morbidity	2.26	181
Total		839
Risk Group 5 (2.49 +)		
Age 41–50, cancer	2.62	8
Age 51–60, diabetes	2.52	280
Age 51–60, collagen disease	3.31	15
Age 51–60, cancer	3.49	20
Age 61–70, social	2.69	5
Age 61–70, other primary	2.80	114
Age 61–70, cardiovascular	2.74	12
Age 61–70, diabetes	3.04	214
Age 61–70, collagen disease	3.98	9
Age 61–70, cancer	4.20	26
Age 71–90, interstitial nephr.	2.75	26
Age 71–90, heart disease	2.91	38
Age 71–90, social	3.78	2
Age 71–90, cardiovascular	3.85	7
Age 71–90, other primary	3.93	63
Age 71–90, diabetes	4.27	65
Age 71–90, collagen disease	5.60	1
Age 71–90, cancer	5.90	16
Total		921

Figure 6
Proportional Hazard Curves

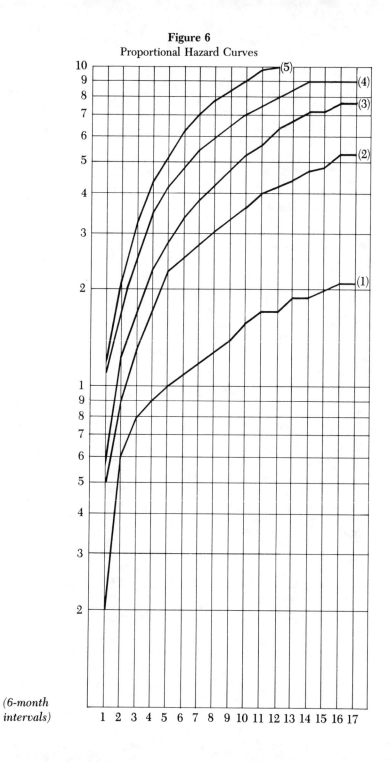

(6-month intervals)

The plots should be roughly parallel. Figure 6 illustrates the plots of the cumulative hazard function for the five risk groups at six-month intervals. The graph suggests that the proportional hazard assumption is reasonable.

Notes

Part I introduction

1. The public sense of medical technology is difficult to assess directly. Few studies consider public expectations for medical technology as an issue, focusing instead on the diffusion of technologies, costs of technology, the assessment of technology, the regulation of technology, or the ethical implications of technology.

Many medical technologies are clearly involved in the intimate interstices of living and dying, but even these are most often considered problems of measurement rather than as personal or cultural experience. See, for example, B. J. McNeil and E. G. Cravalho, eds., *Critical Issues in Medical Technology* (Boston: Auburn House, 1982); S. Altman and R. Blendon, eds., *Medical Technology: The Culprit behind Health Care Costs?* (Washington, D.C.: U.S. Government Printing Office, 1977); or L. Russell, *Technology in Hospitals: Medical Advances and Their Diffusion* (Washington, D.C.: Brookings Institution, 1979).

S. J. Reiser's *Medicine and the Reign of Technology* (New York: Cambridge University Press, 1979) does explore the historical development of medical technology and its influence on the experience of doctors and patients alike. He recognizes that a "mechanical view of human beings" can "inexorably direct the view of both doctor and patient to the measurable aspects of illness [and] away from the human factors" (p. 229).

Most conventional studies of medical technology share Reiser's concerns. An approach to solutions for these and other problems, however, is often sought through the application of additional technologies (from outside medicine). See S. Wolf and B. Berle, *The Technological Imperative in Medicine* (New York: Plenum Press, 1981). For example, a simple solution to

195

the high financial costs of medical technologies and the equally high (but difficult to measure) human costs of such procedures would be to apply the mathematical techniques of formal decision analysis to guide the "rational" use of medical technology. Another example: many doctors do not take good patient histories because of increasing reliance on laboratory tests; this book suggests using history-taking algorithms for computers, transforming a doctor-patient problem into a computer-patient solution.

The cultural experience of technology as a transformation of human relationships is considered in the following general works: L. Mumford, *Technics and Human Development: The Myth of the Machine*, vol. 1 (New York: Harvest Books, 1967); J. Ellul, *The Technological Society* (New York: Vintage Books, 1964); D. Boorstin, *The Republic of Technology* (New York: Harper Colophon, 1978); and D. Nobel, *America by Design* (New York: Oxford University Press, 1979).

2. See, for example, K. Hubner, *Critique of Scientific Reason* (Chicago: University of Chicago Press, 1983). In particular, part 3 of this book considers "The Scientific-Technological World and the Mythological World" (pp. 207–50). See also L. Winner, *Autonomous Technology* (Cambridge: M.I.T. University Press, 1977); T. Kuhn, *The Structure of Scientific Revolutions* (Chicago: University of Chicago Press, 1962); P. Feyerabend, *Against Method* (London: Verson, 1975).

All of these works consider science as deeply rooted in the same politics, biases, and cultural traditions as other human activities. This framework is critical of the common notion of science as an objective domain of reason. There is good and bad science, but value-free inquiry is impossible.

3. The basis for medicine's authority is a complex issue most recently taken up in P. Starr, *The Social Transformation of Medicine* (New York: Basic Books, 1982). In his brief discussion of "cultural authority," Starr recognizes the functional connection between science, technology, and medical authority, but he dismisses too quickly the profound implications of the *ideological* relationship between science and medicine. Of course, the actual contribution of clearly effective, technological therapeutics to medical authority was minimal before 1935. But the belief in science, independent of established effectiveness, was an important component of medical authority: doctors wore the mantle of scientific legitimacy. This authority was itself derived from a deeper level of cultural meaning; see J. Comaroff, "Medicine: Symbol and Ideology," in P. Wright and A. Treacher, eds., *The Problem of Medical Knowledge* (Edinburgh: Edinburgh University Press, 1982).

4. See, for example, B. Ehrenreich and J. Ehrenreich, *The American Health Empire: Power, Profit and Politics* (New York: Vintage Books, 1971); V. Navarro, *Medicine under Capitalism* (Canton, Mass.: Prodist, 1976).

5. E. R. Brown, *Rockefeller Medicine Men: Medicine and Capitalism in America* (Berkeley: University of California Press, 1979); H. Waitzkin and B.

Waterman, *The Exploitation of Illness in Capitalist Society* (Indianapolis: Bobbs-Merrill, 1974).

6. See H. D. Banta and C. J. Behney, "Policy Formation and Technology Assessment," *Milbank Memorial Fund Quarterly: Health and Society* 59 (1981): 445–79; J. B. McKinlay, "From Promising Report to Standard Procedure: Seven Stages in the Career of Medical Innovation," *Milbank Memorial Fund Quarterly: Health and Society* 59, no. 3 (1981): 374–411; H. Waitzkin, "A Marxian Interpretation of the Growth and Development of Coronary Care Technology," *American Journal of Public Health* 69, no. 12(1979): 1260–68.

7. I. K. Zola, "Medicine as an Institution of Social Control," *Sociological Review* N.S. 20 (1972): 487–504.

8. See P. Conrad and R. Kern, *The Sociology of Health and Illness: Critical Perspectives* (New York: St. Martin's Press, 1985); and H. Waitzkin, *The Second Sickness: Contradictions of Capitalist Health Care* (New York: Free Press, 1983).

9. C. Geertz, *The Interpretation of Culture* (New York: Basic Books, 1974).

10. M. Foucault, *The Birth of the Clinic* (New York: Vintage Books, 1975), p. 13.

11. See McKinlay, "From Promising Report to Standard Procedure."

12. J. R. Gusfield, *The Culture of Public Problems* (Chicago: University of Chicago Press, 1981), p. 22.

13. D. Rennie, "Nephrology Comes of Age," *New England Journal of Medicine* 297 (1977): 1461–62.

14. S. Alexander, "They Decide Who Lives and Who Dies: Medical Miracle Puts Moral Burden on Small Committee," *Life* 53 (9 Nov. 1962).

15. R. Fox and J. Swazey, *The Courage to Fail: A Social View of Organ Transplants and Dialysis*, 2nd ed. (Chicago: University of Chicago Press, 1978).

16. B. J. Bernstein, "The Artificial Heart: Is It a Boon or a High-Tech Fix?" *The Nation*, 22 January 1983.

17. A. Anderson, "Dialysis or Death," *New York Times Magazine*, 2 March 1976, pp. 38–41.

18. Ibid., p. 39.

19. Ibid., p. 39.

20. Ibid., p. 40.

21. L. Meyer, "Kidney Care Plan's Cost Soars," *Washington Post*, 19 July 1972, p. A3; R. D. Lyons, "Concern Rising over Costs of Kidney Dialysis Program," *New York Times*, 28 April 1972, p. A16.

22. L. K. Altman, "Transplants Shortage of Donors Still Acute," *New York Times*, 29 May 1977; "Alternatives to Kidney Dialysis," *Wall Street Journal*, Feb.–March 1978.

23. R. Reinhold, "Economics of Life and Death Arises in Debate over Rising Kidney Therapy," *New York Times*, 25 May 1982, pp. C1, C4.

24. Ibid., p. C4.

25. R. A. Gutman, W. N. Stead, and R. R. Robinson, "Physical Activity and Employment Status of Patients on Maintenance Dialysis," *New England Journal of Medicine* 304 (1981): 309–13.

26. P. W. Eggers, *Life Expectancy and Use of Services by Persons with End-Stage Renal Disease Enrolled in Medicare* (Health Care Financing Administration, Office of Research, Dec. 1979).

Chapter 1

1. G. B. Kolata, "Dialysis after Nearly a Decade," *Science* 208 (1980): 473–76.

2. From a personal interview with a federal official, DHEW renal disease section, April 1976.

3. See L. D. Baydin, "The End-Stage Renal Disease Network: An Attempt through Federal Legislation to Regionalize Health Care Delivery," *Medical Care* 15 (July 1977).

4. Examples are such articles as P. G. Jenkins, "Self-Hemodialysis—The Optimum Mode of Dialytic Therapy," *Archives of Internal Medicine*, 136 (1976): 357–61; E. A. Friedman et al., "Pragmatic Realities in Uremia Treatment," *New England Journal of Medicine* 298 (1978): 368–72.

5. J. Merrill, *The Treatment of Renal Failure* (Orlando, Fla.: Grune and Stratton, 1975), p. 81. Also R. Altman, "Sometimes Kidneys Are Transported from Country to Country," *New York Times*, 18 July 1978, p. 34.

6. See R. A. Gutman, W. W. Stead, and R. R. Robinson, "Physical Activity and Employment Status of Patients on Maintenance Dialysis," *New England Journal of Medicine* 304 (1981): 309–13.

7. W. J. Kolf, "Artificial Kidneys in the Seventies," *Nephron* 9 (1972): 276.

8. C. H. Calland, "Iatrogenic Problems in End-Stage Renal Failure," *New England Journal of Medicine* 287 (1974): 334.

9. P. V. Strange and A. T. Sumner, "Predicting Treatment Costs and Life Expectancy for End-Stage Renal Disease," *New England Journal of Medicine* 298 (1978): 372–79. This model, however, presents an overly simplistic approach to ESRD and does not incorporate social factors in the natural history of the disease. More technically correct approaches to survival analysis include: T. A. Hutchinson, D. E. Thomas, B. McGibbon, "Predicting Survival in Adults with End-Stage Renal Disease: An Age Equivalence Index," *Annals of Internal Medicine* 96 (1982): 417–23; J. M. Weller, E. K. Port, R. D. Swartz, et al., "Analysis of Survival of End-Stage Renal Disease Patients," *Kidney International* 21 (1982): 78–83.

10. R. A. Rettig and E. L. Marks, *Implementing the End-Stage Renal Disease Program of Medicare* (Santa Monica, Cal.: Rand Corporation, Sept. 1980).

11. D. Rennie, "Nephrology Comes of Age," *New England Journal of Medicine* 297 (1977): 1461–62. Rennie argues that the development of the technology of dialysis vitalized this marginal clinical specialty.

12. Ibid., p. 1461 (emphasis added).

13. Ibid., p. 1462 (emphasis added).

14. B. Burton, ed., "Advances in Dialysis: A Symposium," *Clinical Nephrology* 9, no. 4 (1978).

15. H. Marks, "Medical Science and Clinical Ambiguity: The Role of Clinical Trials in Therapeutic Controversies" (Harvard University School of Public Health, Center for the Analysis of Health Practices, Nov. 1981).

16. S. Klahr, K. Nolf, and R. Luke, *End-Stage Renal Disease: Pathophysiology, Dialysis, and Transplantation*, National Center for Health Care Technology Monograph Series (Washington, D.C., May 1981).

17. E. Lowrie and C. Hampers, "Proprietary Dialysis and the End Stage Renal Disease Program," *Dialysis and Transplantation* 11, no. 3 (March 1982).

18. H. Krakuer et al., "The Recent U.S. Experience in the Treatment of Endstage Renal Disease by Dialysis and Transplantation," *New England Journal of Medicine* 308 (1983): 1558–63.

19. Klahr, Nolf, and Luke, *End-Stage Renal Disease*, p. 24.

20. Ibid., p. 31.

21. P. Eggers, R. Connerton, and M. McMullan, "The Medicare Experience with End-stage Renal Disease: Trends in Incidence, Prevalence, and Survival," *Health Care Financing Review* 5, vol. 3 (Spring 1984): 69–88.

22. A. S. Relman and D. Rennie, "Treatment of End-Stage Renal Disease: Free but Not Equal," *New England Journal of Medicine* 303 (1980): 996–98.

23. C. Blagg, "Cui Bono?: A Response to Drs. Hampers and Hager," *Dialysis and Transplantation* 8 (1979): 501–13.

24. Lowrie and Hampers, "Proprietary Dialysis," p. 201.

25. See note 4, above.

26. For example, see G. M. Abbey, vice-president, Travenol Laboratories, Inc., Hearing before the Subcommittee on Oversight of the Committee on Ways and Means, House of Representatives, 97th Cong., 2nd sess., serial 97-59 (22 April 1982), pp. 252–59.

27. Krakuer et al., "Recent U.S. Experience," p. 1562.

28. C. K. Davis, administrator, HCFA, DHHS, Hearing before the Subcommittee on Oversight of the Committee on Ways and Means, House of Representatives, 97th Cong., 2nd sess., serial 97-59 (22 April 1982), pp. 171–213.

29. W. Vollmer, P. Wahl, and C. Blagg, "Survival with Dialysis and Transplantation in Patients with End-Stage Renal Disease," *New England Journal of Medicine* 38 (1983): 1555.

30. J. Prottas, "Encouraging Altruism: Public Attitudes and the Marketing of Organ Donations," *Millbank Memorial Fund Quarterly* 61, no. 2 (1983): 278–306.

31. Ibid., p. 302.

32. W. B. Stason and B. A. Barnes, *Effectiveness and Costs of Continuous Ambulatory Peritoneal Dialysis*, Office of Technology Assessment, Congress of the United States (Washington, D.C.: Government Printing Office, Sept. 1985).

Chapter 2

1. The data in this and the next chapter are based on a two-year study of an end-stage renal disease treatment program at an urban teaching hospital affiliated with a major medical school. The study employed a range of methodologies including participant observation, structured interviews, informal semistructured interviews, and a detailed analysis of the medical record of patients treated in the unit. Patients, members of their families, staff, and other hospital personnel were the subjects of this study. Quotations from staff meetings and interviews were tape recorded and later transcribed. The medical records of all patients were abstracted with particular attention paid to nursing notes and consultant notes (e.g., psychiatry). The names of all participants in this study will remain confidential as will the name of the hospital.

Is this a "representative sample" of ESRD treatment? I believe that this sample reflects the range of problems experienced in the treatment of this catastrophic illness. Of course not every treatment program will have experienced exactly the same type of problems discussed in this chapter but they will have experienced similar decisions, choices, and dilemmas. Some of these experiences become part of the routine of daily life in the ESRD clinic. For example, a study published in 1986 found that over 20 percent of deaths in a renal unit resulted from a decision to "pull the plug." This chapter presents the social context behind these adverse clinical outcomes.

2. All quotations in this section have been derived from interviews, informal discussions, and taped observations of staff members and patients in this program. Some information also derives from abstracts of particular patients' medical records and will be labeled as such in the text. To footnote each entry would tend to confuse the reader more than to clarify.

Chapter 3

1. E. M. Gerson, "The Social Character of Illness: Deviance or Politics?" *Social Science and Medicine* 10 (1976): 219–24.

2. A. Strauss, *Chronic Illness and the Quality of Life* (St. Louis: C. V. Mosby, 1975), p. 149.

3. See, for example, R. C. Fox and J. P. Swazey, *The Courage to Fail: A Social View of Organ Transplants and Dialysis* (Chicago: University of Chicago Press, 1974; 2nd ed., 1978); R. G. Simmons, S. D. Klein, and R. L. Simmons, *Gift of Life: The Social and Psychological Impact of Organ Transplantation* (New York: John Wiley, 1977); J. W. Czaczkes and A. Kaplan-DeNour, *Chronic Hemodialysis as a Way of Life* (New York: Brunner/Mazel, 1978).

4. See B. T. Burton, "The Federal Government's Role in the Management of End-Stage Renal Disease," *Kidney International* Supplement 8 (June 1978): 61–84; and R. W. Evans, C. R. Blegg, and F. A. Bryan, Jr., "Implications for Health Care Policy: A Social and Demographic Profile of Hemodialysis Patients in the U.S.," *Journal of the American Medical Association*, 245, no. 5 (6 Feb. 1981): 487–91.

5. Simmons et al., *Gift of Life*; R. Gokal et al., "Continuous Ambulatory Peritoneal Dialysis: One Year's Experience in a U.K. Dialysis Unit," *British Medical Journal* 281, no. 6238 (6 Aug. 1980): 474–77; M. E. O'Brien, *The Courage to Survive: The Life Career of the Chronic Dialysis Patient* (Orlando, Fla.: Grune and Stratton, 1983).

6. Czaczkes and Kaplan-DeNour, *Chronic Hemodialysis*; Simmons et al., *Gift of Life*.

7. W. B. Stason and B. A. Barnes, *Effectiveness and Costs of Continuous Ambulatory Peritoneal Dialysis*, Office of Technology Assessment, Congress of the United States (Washington, D.C.: Government Printing Office, Sept. 1985).

8. Strauss, *Chronic Illness*, p. 23.

9. Ibid., p. 35.

10. See Czaczkes and Kaplan-DeNour, *Chronic Hemodialysis*, p. 146; I. S. Halper, "Psychiatric Observations in a Chronic Hemodialysis Program," *Symposium on Diseases of the Kidney*, Medical Clinics of North America 55, no. 1 (Jan. 1972): 177–91; D. Anger and D. W. Anger, "Dialysis Ambivalence: A Matter of Life and Death," *American Journal of Nursing* 76, no. 2 (1976): 276–77; O'Brien, *Courage to Survive*, pp. 11–42.

11. J. C. Nemiah, *Foundations of Psychopathology* (New York: Oxford University Press, 1961), p. 309.

12. Fox and Swazey, *Courage to Fail*, pp. 11–42.

13. Ibid., p. 102.

14. R. A. Rettig and E. L. Marks, *Implementing the End-Stage Renal Disease Program of Medicare* (Santa Monica, Cal.: Rand Corporation, 1980).

15. A. Kaplan-DeNour, "Psychotherapy with Patients on Chronic Hemodialysis," *American Journal of Psychiatry* 116 (1970): 207–15; M. Viederman, "Adaptive and Maladaptive Regression in Hemodialysis," *Psychiatry* 37 (Feb. 1974): 68–77; G. M. Devins et al., "Helplessness and

Depression in End-Stage Renal Disease," *Journal of Abnormal Psychology* 90 (1981): 531–45.

16. C. H. Calland, "Iatrogenic Problems in End-Stage Renal Failure," *New England Journal of Medicine* 287 (1974): 334–36.

17. Simmons et al., *Gift of Life*.

18. Fox and Swazey, *Courage to Fail*, p. 9.

19. Czaczkes and Kaplan-DeNour, *Chronic Hemodialysis*.

20. Halper, "Psychiatric Observations"; O'Brien, *Courage to Survive*.

21. Anger and Anger, "Dialysis Ambivalence," p. 276.

22. Simmons et al., *Gift of Life*.

23. Ibid., pp. 383–85.

24. O'Brien, *Courage to Survive*, p. 48.

25. F. O. Finkelstein, S. H. Finkelstein, and T. E. Steele, "Assessment of Marital Relationships of Hemodialysis Patients," *American Journal of the Medical Sciences* 271, no. 1 (1976): 21–28. Also G. D. Chowanec and Y. M. Binik, "End Stage Renal Disease and the Marital Dyad: A Literature Review and Critique," *Social Science and Medicine* 16 (1982): 1551–58.

26. C. S. Santopietro, "Meeting the Emotional Needs of Hemodialysis Patients and Their Spouses," *American Journal of Nursing* 4 (April 1975): 629–32.

27. D. B. Fishman and C. J. Schneider, "Predicting Emotional Adjustment in Home Dialysis Patients and Their Relatives," *Journal of Chronic Disease* 25 (1972): 99–109.

28. Halper, "Psychiatric Observations"; Kaplan-DeNour, "Psychotherapy with Patients on Chronic Hemodialysis"; Czaczkes and DeNour, *Chronic Hemodialysis*; H. S. Abram and D. C. Buchanon, "The Gift of Life: A Review of the Psychological Aspects of Kidney Transplantation," *International Journal of Psychiatry in Medicine* 7, no. 2 (1976–77): 153–54; L. E. Lancaster and P. Pierce, "Total Body Manifestation of End-Stage Renal Disease and Related Medical and Nursing Management," in L. E. Lancaster, ed., *The Patient with End-Stage Renal Disease* (New York: Wiley, 1979), pp. 1–60.

29. H. S. Abram, "The Psychiatrist, the Treatment of Chronic Renal Failure and the Prolongation of Life: III," *American Journal of Psychiatry* 128, no. 12 (June 1972): 1534–39.

30. J. J. VanLeeuwen and D. E. Matthews, "Comprehensive Mental Health Care in a Pediatric Dialysis-Transplantation Program," *Canadian Medical Association Journal* 113 (22 Nov. 1975): 959–62.

31. R. G. Wright, F. Sand, and G. Livingston, "Psychological Stress during Hemodialysis for Chronic Renal Failure," *Annals of Internal Medicine* 64 (1966): 611–21; also M. E. O'Brian, "Effective Social Environment and Hemodialysis Adaptation: A Panel Analysis," *Journal of Health & Social Behavior* 21 (1980): 360–70.

32. Halper, "Psychiatric Observations," p. 189.

33. H. S. Abrams, "Psychiatric Reflections Adaptation to Repetitive Dialysis, *Kidney International* 6 (1974): 67–72.

34. Halper, "Psychiatric Observations," p. 184.

35. Calland, "Iatrogenic Problems," p. 335.

36. Ibid., p. 335.

37. Abram and Buchanon, "Gift of Life."

38. R. A. Gutman, W. W. Stead, and R. R. Robinson, "Physical Activity and Employment Status of Patients on Maintenance Dialysis," *New England Journal of Medicine* 304 (1981): 309–13.

Chapter 4

1. D. Armstrong, *Political Anatomy of the Body: Medical Knowledge in Britain in the Twentieth Century* (Cambridge: Cambridge University Press, 1983); E. J. Cassel, "The Nature of Suffering and the Goals of Medicine," *New England Journal of Medicine* 306 (1983): 639–46; N. Cousins, *Anatomy of an Illness as Perceived by the Patient* (New York, W. W. Norton, 1979): E. G. Mishier, L. R. Amara Singham, S. T. Houser, R. Liem, S. D. Osherson, and N. E. Waxler, *Social Contexts of Health, Illness, and Patient Care* (Cambridge: Cambridge University Press, 1981); S. Sontag, *Illness as Metaphor* (New York: Farrar, Straus, and Giroux, 1977); M. T. Taussig, "Reification and the Consciousness of the Patient," *Social Science and Medicine* 14B (1980): 3–13.

2. An anthropological analysis of "joking relationships" can be found in A. R. Radcliffe-Brown, "On Joking Relationships," in *Structure and Function in Primitive Societies* (New York: Free Press, 1965). These relationships "only exist between individuals or groups which are in some way socially separated" (p. 104). See also J. Emerson, "Behavior in Private Places: Sustaining Definitions of Reality in Gynecological Examinations," in H. P. Drietzel, ed., *Patterns of Communicative Behavior* (New York: Macmillan, 1970), pp. 73–101.

3. M. B. Scott and S. M. Lyman, "Accounts," *American Sociological Review* 46, no. 1 (1968): 46–62; C. W. Mills, "Situated Actions and Vocabularies of Motive," *American Sociological Review* 5, no. 3 (1940): 904–13.

Part II introduction

1. See, for example, J. B. Gross, W. E. Keane, and A. K. McDonald, "Survival and Rehabilitation of Patients on Home Hemodialysis: Five Years' Experience," *Annals of Internal Medicine* 78 (1973): 341–46; M. R. Higgins, M. Grace, and J. B. Dossetor, "Survival of Patients Treated for End-Stage Renal Disease by Dialysis and Transplantation," *Canadian Medical Associa-*

tion Journal 117 (1977): 880–83; and J. M. Weller, F. K. Port, R. D. Swartz, et al., "Analysis of Survival of End-stage Renal Disease Patients," *Kidney International* 21 (1982): 78–83.

2. A. S. Relman and D. Rennie, "Treatment of End-Stage Renal Disease, Free but Not Equal," *New England Journal of Medicine* 303 (1980): 996–97.

3. R. A. Rettig and E. L. Marks, *Implementing the End-Stage Renal Disease Program of Medicare* (Santa Monica, Cal.: Rand Corporation, Sept. 1980).

4. A. Plough, "Medical Technology and the Crisis of Experience: The Cost of Clinical Legitimation," *Social Science and Medicine* 15F (1981): 89–101.

Chapter 5

1. *Prevalence of Chronic Condition in the United States*, Vital and Health Statistics, Series 10 (1979).

2. H. Birnbaum, *The Cost of Catastrophic Illness* (Lexington, Mass.: D. C. Heath, 1977).

3. Comptroller General of the United States, *Treatment of Chronic Kidney Failure: Dialysis, Transplant Costs, and the Need for More Vigorous Efforts* (Washington, D.C.: Government Printing Office, 25 June 1975), pp. 38–39.

4. W. B. Stason and B. A. Barnes, *Effectiveness and Costs of Continuous Ambulatory Peritoneal Dialysis*, Office of Technology Assessment, Congress of the United States (Washington, D.C.: Government Printing Office, Sept. 1985).

5. A. Plough and M. Shwartz, "Prospective Models for Medical Technology Assessment" (Waltham, Mass.: University Health Policy Consortium, 1980).

6. S. Alexander, "They Decide Who Lives and Who Dies," *Life* 53 (9 Nov. 1962): 102–4ff.

7. B. T. Burton, *Kidney Disease Program Analysis: A Report to the Surgeon General*, U.S. Department of Health, Education, and Welfare, Public Health Service (Washington, D.C.: Government Printing Office, 1967).

8. C. W. Gottschalk, *Report of the Committee on Chronic Disease*, U.S. Bureau of the Budget (Washington, D.C.: Government Printing Office, 1967).

9. Hearings on National Health Insurance Proposals before the House Committee on Ways and Means, 92nd Cong., 1st sess., 1971, pt. 7, pp. 1524–46.

10. J. K. Ingelhart, "Playing the Role of Doctor," *National Journal*, 14 May 1977.

11. Hearings on Medicare's End-Stage Renal Disease Program before the Committee on Oversight of the House Committee on Ways and Means, 92nd Cong., 1st sess., 1975, pp. 1–150.

12. U.S. Congress, House of Representatives, Committee on Ways and Means, *Background Information on Kidney Disease Benefits under Medicare*, 94th Cong., 1st sess., 24 June 1975, Committee Print.

13. P. A. Hoffstein, K. I. Krueger, and R. J. Wineman, "Dialysis Costs: Results of a Diverse Sample Study," *Kidney International* 9 (1976): 286–93.

14. S. D. Roberts, T. L. Gross, and D. R. Maxwell, "Cost-Effective Care of End-Stage Renal Disease: A Billion Dollar Question," *Annals of Internal Medicine* 92, no. 2, pt. 1 (1980): 243–48.

15. E. Bergsten et al., "A Study of Patients on Chronic Hemodialysis," *Scandinavian Journal of Social Medicine* 11 (1977): 1.

16. B. A. Barnes, "Current Status of Home Dialysis and Related Issues Based on Literature Review of 1977, 1978" (Center for the Analysis of Health Practice, Harvard University, 1979).

17. P.L. 95-292, 95th Cong., 13 June 1978.

Chapter 6

1. National Medical Care, Inc., *Annual Report—1976* (Brookline, Mass., 1975).

2. I. Illich, *Medical Nemesis* (New York: Pantheon, 1976); M. Renaud, "Structural Constraints to State Intervention in Health," *International Journal of Health Services* 5 (1975): 559.

3. "The Burgeoning Business in Artificial Kidneys," *Duns Review*, Oct. 1971, pp. 81–84.

4. Frost and Sullivan, *Analysis of the Market for Dialysis Equipment and Supplies* (New York: n. pub., 1977 and 1981).

5. D. A. Pearson, J. D. Thompson, and T. J. Stranova, "Patient and Program Costs Associated with Chronic Hemodialysis Care," *Inquiry* 13 (March 1976): 23–28. See also A. T. Romeo, *The Hemodialysis Equipment and Disposables Industry*, Office of Technology Assessment, Congress of the United States (Washington, D.C.: Government Printing Office, Dec. 1984).

6. "Growth Expected for Baxter," *Wall Street Journal*, 17 March 1976, p. 14.

7. Baxter Laboratories, Inc., *Annual Report—1976* (Deerfield, Ill., 1975), p. 14.

8. "Baxter Travenol Labs' Outlook," *Wall Street Journal*, 6 May 1976, sec. 4, p. 26.

9. Securities and Exchange Commission, *Form 10-K: Baxter Laboratories, Inc.*, 31 Dec. 1975.

10. C. Elia, "Heard on the Street: Hospital Supply Profits," *Wall Street Journal*, 19 Dec. 1974, sec. 3, p. 31.

11. Ibid., p. 31.

12. Baxter, *Annual Report*, p. 21.

13. *Form 10-K: Baxter*, p. 16.

14. "U.S. Drug Makers Flock to Ireland," *Wall Street Journal*, 31 March 1975, p. 8.

15. Baxter, *Annual Report*, p. 17.

16. "Baxter Labs Admits Foreign Payments of Over $2.1 Million," *Wall Street Journal*, 24 Feb. 1976, sec. 2, p. 2.

17. Baxter, *Annual Report*, p. 99.

18. "Vernitron Corp. Agrees to Settle Patent Suit Brought by Baxter Labs," *Wall Street Journal*, 13 Feb. 1976, sec. 3, p. 4.

19. *Form 10-K: Baxter*, p. 18.

20. Baxter, *Annual Report*, p. 11.

21. Ibid., p. 12.

22. Ibid., p. 13.

23. "Baxter Travenol Labs' Outlook," *Wall Street Journal*, 6 May 1976, sec. 4, p. 26.

24. "The Money in Hospital Throwaways," *Commercial and Financial Chronicle*, 22 April 1974, pp. 128–29.

25. "The Burgeoning Business in Artificial Kidneys," *Duns Review*, Oct. 1971, pp. 81–84.

26. National Medical Care, Inc., *Annual Report—1978* (Brookline, Mass., 1979).

27. Ibid.

28. D. Bird, "Doctor Who Runs Chain of Dialysis Centers Trying, with State Senator's Aid, to Get a City Contract," *New York Times*, 29 Sept. 1975, sec. 1, p. 25.

29. Ibid.

30. National Medical Care, *Annual Report—1976*.

31. Ibid., p. B-2.

32. "National Medical Care Sees Rise in 1976 Net," *Wall Street Journal*, 4 Oct. 1976, sec. 2, p. 7.

33. Securities and Exchange Commission, *Form 10-K: National Medical Care, Inc.*, 31 Dec. 1976.

34. Ibid., p. 6.

35. National Medical Care, *Annual Report—1976*, p. 7.

36. Ibid., p. 6.

37. Ibid., p. 11.

38. Ibid., p. 22.

39. Ibid., p. 14 (emphasis added).

40. G. B. Kolata, "NMC Thrives Selling Dialysis," *Science* 208 (1980): 379–80; G. B. Kolata, "Dialysis after Nearly a Decade," *Science* 208 (1980): 473–76; also Securities and Exchange Commission, *Form 10-K; National Medical Care, Inc.*, 31 Dec. 1979.

41. Securities and Exchange Commission, *Form 10-K; National Medical Care, Inc.*, 31 Dec. 1979.

42. Frost and Sullivan, *Analysis of the Market*, p. 119.

43. Department of Health and Human Services, HCFA, "Medicare Program; End-Stage Renal Disease Program: Prospective Reimbursement for Dialysis Services," Part IV, *Federal Register* 47, no. 30 (12 Feb. 1982).

44. A. B. Fisher, "Washington Reins In the Dialysis Business," *Fortune*, 25 July 1983, pp. 67–69.

45. W. B. Stason and B. A. Barnes, *Effectiveness and Costs of Continuous Ambulatory Peritoneal Dialysis*, Office of Technology Assessment, Congress of the United States (Washington, D.C.: Government Printing Office, Sept. 1985), p. 7.

46. B. A. Mohl, "Dialysis: Life and Death Business," *Boston Globe*, 24 May 1983, p. 53.

47. Fisher, "Washington," p. 68.

48. R. Brammer, "Problems at Delmed," *Barron's*, 23 April 1984, p. 2. Also, "Delmed Objects to Story in Barron's," *Barron's*, 30 April 1984, p. 4.

49. D. French, "Barron's Story Elicits Angry Reply by Delmed," *Boston Globe*, 24 April 1984, p. 35.

50. Brammer, "Problems at Delmed."

51. National Medical Care, *Annual Report—1983*, p. 10.

52. Ibid., p. 6.

53. Ibid.

54. A. Bernstein, "J. Peter Grace Is Swallowing His Pride and Shifting Course—Well, Sort Of," *Business Week*, Dec. 10, 1984, p. 99.

Chapter 7

1. R. A. Rettig and E. L. Marks, *Implementing the End-Stage Renal Disease Program of Medicare* (Santa Monica, Cal.: Rand Corporation, Sept. 1980).

2. Department of Health and Human Services, HCFA, "Medicare Program; End-Stage Renal Disease Program: Prospective Reimbursement for Dialysis Services," Part IV, *Federal Register* 47, no. 30 (12 Feb. 1982).

3. D. S. Greenberg, "Renal Politics—Washington Report," *New England Journal of Medicine* 298, no. 25 (22 June 1978): 1427–28; E. Lowrie and C. Hampers, "The Success of Medicare's End-Stage Renal Disease Program: The Case for Profits and the Private Marketplace," *New England Journal of Medicine* 305 (1981): 434–38; P. W. Eggers, "Analyses of Indicators of Case-Mix Differences between Free-Standing Facility and Hospital-Based Medicare ESRD Patients," Working Paper #OR38 (Health Care Financing Administration, Office of Research and Demonstration, 1982).

4. HCFA, "Medicare Program."

5. Quoted in A. B. Fisher, "Washington Reins In the Dialysis Business," *Fortune*, 25 July 1983, p. 69.

6. G. B. Kolata, "NMC Thrives Selling Dialysis," *Science* 208 (1980): 379–80.

7. A. S. Relman, "The New Medical Industrial Complex," *New England Journal of Medicine* 303 (1980): 963–70.

8. Ibid., p. 963.

9. Ibid., p. 969.

10. A. S. Relman and D. Rennie, "Treatment of End-Stage Renal Disease: Free but Not Equal," *New England Journal of Medicine* 303 (1980): 996–98.

11. Ibid., p. 998.

12. Greenberg, "Renal Politics—Washington Report," pp. 1427–28.

13. Rettig and Marks, *Implementing the End-Stage Renal Disease Program*.

14. J. Prottas, "Retreat to Regulation, Administration of the End-Stage Renal Disease Program" (Waltham, Mass.: University Health Policy Consortium, 1982).

15. Ibid., p. 25.

16. Lowrie and Hampers, "The Success of Medicare's End-Stage Renal Disease Program," pp. 434–38.

17. Quoted in Fisher, "Washington Reins In the Dialysis Business," p. 69.

18. Lowrie and Hampers, "The Success of Medicare's End-Stage Renal Disease Program," pp. 434–38.

19. Ibid., p. 435.

20. Ibid., p. 438.

21. Ibid., p. 436.

22. C. R. Blagg, "Profits and the End-Stage Renal Disease Program," *New England Journal of Medicine* 306 (1983): 369–70; A. P. Ludin and E. A. Friedman, "Letter," in ibid., p. 370; V. W. Sidel, "Letter," in ibid.; J. D. Fett, "Letter," in ibid.

23. E. W. Lowrie and C. L. Hampers, "Response," in ibid., pp. 370–71.

24. Ibid., p. 371.

25. Fisher, "Washington Reins In the Dialysis Business," p. 68.

26. Ibid., p. 69.

27. See the review of CAPD in W. B. Stason and B. A. Barnes, *Effectiveness and Costs of Continuous Ambulatory Peritoneal Dialysis*, Office of Technology Assessment, Congress of the United States (Washington, D.C.: Government Printing Office, Sept. 1985).

28. HCFA, "Medicare Program."

29. Ibid.

30. Lowrie and Hampers, "The Case for Profits"; Eggers, "Analyses of Indicators of Case-Mix Differences."

31. A. R. Feinstein, "The Pretherapeutic Classification of Comorbidity in Chronic Disease," *Journal of Chronic Disease* 23 (1970): 455–68; T. A. Hutchinson, D. C. Thomas, and B. MacGibbon, "Predicting Survival in Adults with End-Stage Renal Disease: An Age Equivalence Index," *Annals of Internal Medicine* 96 (1982): 417–423; M. A. Kaplan and A. R. Feinstein, "The Importance of Classifying Initial Comorbidity in Evaluating the Outcome of Diabetes Mellitus," *Journal of Chronic Disease* 27 (1974): 387–404.

32. A. L. Plough and S. R. Salem, "Social and Contextual Factors in the Analysis of Mortality in End-Stage Renal Disease Patients: Implications for Health Policy," *American Journal of Public Health* 72 (1982): 1293–95.

33. E. G. Lowrie and C. L. Hampers, "Proprietary Dialysis and the ESRD Program," *Dialysis and Transplantation* 11, no. 3 (March 1982): 191–204.

34. A. L. Plough, S. R. Salem, M. Shwartz, et al., "Case-Mix in End-Stage Renal Disease: Difference between Patients in Hospital-Based and Free-Standing Treatment Facilities," *New England Journal of Medicine* 310 (1984): 1432–36.

35. L. J. Tell, "Volatile Reaction: A Scholarly Study Provokes National Medical Care,"*Barron's*, 18 June 1984, p. 7.

Epilogue

1. E. Stark, "What Is Medicine," *Radical Science Journal* 12 (1982): 47–89.

2. See J. Habermas, *Legitimation Crisis* (Boston: Beacon Press, 1975); A. Gouldner, *The Dialectic of Ideology and Technology* (New York: Oxford University Press, 1982); L. Winner, *Autonomous Technology* (Boston: M.I.T. Press, 1977).

3. See P. Starr, *The Social Transformation of American Medicine* (New York: Basic Books, 1982).

4. L. Winner, *Autonomous Technology*, p. 317.

Appendix

1. D. R. Cox, "Regression Models and Life Tables," *Journal of the Royal Statistical Society* ser. B 34 (1972): 187–220.

2. T. A. Hutchinson, D. C. Thomas, and B. MacGibbon, "Predicting Survival in Adults with End-Stage Renal Disease: An Age Equivalence Index," *Annals of Internal Medicine* 96 (1982): 417–23.

3. R. Kay, "Proportional Hazard Regression Models and the Analysis of Censored Data," *Applied Statistics* 26 (1977): 227–37.

Index